D1074870

The International Review of Child Neurology

Alternating Hemiplegia
of Childhood

The International Review of Child Neurology

The International Review of Child Neurology

Alternating Hemiplegia of Childhood

Editors

Frederick Andermann, M.D., F.R.C.P. (c)

Professor of Neurology and Pediatrics
Departments of Neurology, Neurosurgery and Pediatrics
McGill University
Director, Epilepsy Service
Montreal Neurological Hospital
Montreal, Quebec, Canada

Jean Aicardi, M.D., F.R.C.P.

Honorary Professor of Child Neurology
Institute of Child Health
University of London
London, England

Federico Vigevano, M.D.

Professor of Neurology
Department of Paediatric Neurology
Head, Section of Neurophysiology
"Bambino Gesù" Children's Hospital
Rome, Italy

RAVEN PRESS **NEW YORK**

Raven Press, Ltd., 1185 Avenue of the Americas, New York, New York 10036

Made in the United States of America

Library of Congress Cataloging-in-Publication Data

Alternating hemiplegia of childhood / editors, Frederick Andermann,
    Jean Aicardi, Federico Vigevano.
            p.   cm.
    Includes bibliographical references and index.
    ISBN 0-7817-0163-5
    1. Alternating hemiplegia of childhood.   I. Andermann, Frederick.
II. Aicardi, Jean.   III. Vigevano, Federico.
    [DNLM: 1. Hemiplegia—in infancy & childhood.]
RJ496.A53A45   1994
618.92′83–dc20
DNLM/DLC
for Library of Congress   94-16893

The material contained in this volume was submitted as previously unpublished material, except in the instances in which credit has been given to the source from which some of the illustrative material was derived.

Great care has been taken to maintain the accuracy of the information contained in the volume. However, neither Raven Press nor the editors can be held responsible for errors or for any consequences arising from the use of the information contained herein.

9   8   7   6   5   4   3   2   1

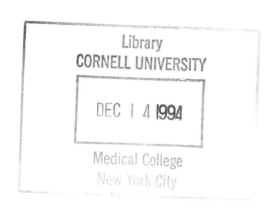

To
the memory of my parents Anny and Adolf,
to my wife Eva,
our son Mark, and
our daughters Lisa and Anne,
who are in turn starting out on the path of inquiry.

F. A.

To
my wife Sandra,
and
our children Cecilia, Andrea, and Giorgio.

F. V.

Contents

Clinical Delineation of the Syndrome

Investigation of Patients with Alternating Hemiplegia of Childhood

Conclusions

Contributing Authors

Jean Aicardi, M.D., F.R.C.P.
Honorary Professor of Child Neurology
Institute of Child Health
University of London
Mecklenburgh Square
London WC1N 2AP, England

Eva Andermann, M.D., Ph.D.
Head, Neurogenetics Unit
Department of Neurology and
*   Neurosurgery*
McGill University
Montreal Neurological Hospital and
*   Institute*
3801 University Street
Montreal, Quebec, H3A 2B4 Canada

Frederick Anderman, M.D.,
F.R.C.P.(C)
Professor of Neurology and Pediatrics
Department of Neurology and
*   Neurosurgery*
McGill University
Director, Epilepsy Service
Montreal Neurological Hospital and
*   Institute*
3801 University Street
Montreal, Quebec, H3A 2B4 Canada

Douglas L. Arnold, M.D.
Associate Professor of Neurology
Department of Neurology and
*   Neurosurgery*
McGill University
Montreal Neurological Hospital and
*   Institute*
3801 University Street
Montreal, Quebec, H3A 2B4 Canada

Andrea Bartuli, M.D.
Section of Metabolic Diseases
"Bambino Gesù" Children's Hospital
Piazza S. Onofrio, 4
00165 Rome, Italy

Peter S. Baxter, M.A., M.D.,
M.R.C.P., D.C.H.
Consultant Paediatrician
Paediatric Neurologist
Department of Paediatrics
Northern General Hospital NHS Trust
Herries Road
Sheffield, S5 7AU England

Laurence Edward Becker, M.D.,
F.R.C.P.(C)
Professor of Pathology and Pediatrics
Department of Pathology
The Hospital for Sick Children
555 University Avenue
Toronto, Ontario, M5G 1X8 Canada

Enrico Bertini, M.D.
Section of Neurophysiology
"Bambino Gesù" Children's Hospital
Piazza S. Onofrio, 4
00165 Rome, Italy

Marie Bourgeois, M.D.
Department of Pediatrics
Hôpital des Enfants Malades
149 rue de Sèvres
75743 Paris Cedex 15 France

Peter R. Camfield, M.D.,
F.R.C.P.(C)
Professor of Pediatrics
Department of Pediatrics
P.O. Box 3070
Dalhousie University
Halifax, Nova Scotia, B3J 3G9 Canada

Vito Colamaria, M.D.
Cattedra di Neuropsichiatria Infantile
Policlinico Borgo Roma
37134 Verona, Italy

Raffaella Cusmai, M.D.
Post Doctoral Fellow
Section of Neurophysiology
"Bambino Gesù" Children's Hospital
Piazza S. Onofrio, 4
00165 Rome, Italy

Bernardo Dalla Bernardina
Cattedra di Neuropsichiatria Infantile
Policlinico Borgo Roma
37134 Verona, Italy

Francesca Darra, M.D.
Cattedra di Neuropsichiatria Infantile
Policlinico Borgo Roma
37134 Verona, Italy

Fernando Dangond, M.D.
Department of Neurology
Brigham and Women's Hospital
Harvard Medical School
Boston, Massachusettes 02115

Nicola De Stefano, M.D.
Post Doctoral Research Fellow
Magnetic Resonance Spectroscopy Unit
Montreal Neurological Hospital and
Institute
3801 University Street
Montreal, Quebec, H3A 2B4 Canada

Matteo Di Capua. M.D.
Section of Neurophysiology
"Bambino Gesù" Children's Hospital
Piazza S. Onofrio, 4
00165 Rome, Italy

Kevin Farrell, M.B., F.R.C.P.(C),
F.R.C.P.(A)
Associate Professor of Neurology
Division of Neurology
Department of Pediatrics
University of British Columbia
British Columbia Children's Hospital
4480 Oak Street
Vancouver, British Columbia, V6H 3V4
Canada

Alan J. Fischman, M.D., Ph.D.
Professor of Radiology
Department of Radiology
Harvard Medical School
Massachusetts General Hospital
32 Fruit Street
Boston, Massachusetts 02114

Elena Fontana, M.D.
Cattedra di Neuropsichiatria Infantile
Policlinico Borgo Roma
37134 Verona, Italy

Anna Franco, M.D.
Cattedra di Neuropsichiatria Infantile
Policlinico Borgo Roma
37134 Verona, Italy

Lucia Fusco, M.D., Ph.D.
Consultant Neurologist
Section of Neurophysiology
"Bambino Gesù" Children's Hospital
Piazza S. Onofrio, 4
00165 Rome, Italy

D. Gardner-Medwin, M.D.,
F.R.C.P.
Consultant Paediatric Neurologist
Newcastle General Hospital
Westgate Road
Newcastle upon Tyne, NE4 6BE England

Licia Giardina, M.D.
Cattedra di Neuropsichiatria Infantile
Policlinico Borgo Roma
37134 Verona, Italy

Françoise Goutières, M.D.
Department of Pediatrics
Hôpital des Enfants Malades
149 rue de Sèvres
75743 Paris Cedex 15, France

Stuart H. Green, M.A., M.B.,
B.Chir., F.R.C.P.
Senior Lecturer
Consultant Paediatric Neurologist
Institute of Child Health
Medical School
University of Birmingham
Birmingham, B16 8ET England

Yvonne M. Hart, M.D., M.R.C.P.
Consultant Neurologist
Department of Neurology
Atkinson Morley's Hospital
Copse Hill
Wimbledon, London, SW20 ONE England

Katsuhiro Kobayashi, M.D.
Department of Child Neurology
Okayama University Medical School
5-1, Shikatacho-2 chome
Okayama, 700, Japan

Simon D. Levin, M.B.Ch.B.,
   F.R.C.P.(E), F.R.C.P.(C)
Assistant Professor of Paediatrics
Department of Paediatrics
University of Western Ontario
800 Commissioners Road East
London, Ontario, N6C 2V5 Canada

Mohamad A. Mikati, M.D.
Associate Professor of Neurology
Director of Epilepsy Research and
   Clinical Neuropharmacology
Department of Neurology
Children's Hospital
Harvard Medical School
300 Longwood Avenue
Boston, Massachusetts 02115

Alessandra Montagnini, M.D.
Cattedra di Neuropsichiatria Infantile
Policlinico Borgo Roma
37134 Verona, Italy

Celia Moss, D.M., M.R.C.P.
Consultant Dermatologist
Department of Dermatology
Birmingham Children's Hospital
Ladywood Middleway
Birmingham, B16 8ET England

Soňa Nevšímalová, M.D. , D.Sc.
Associate Professor of Neurology
Department of Neurology
First Medical Faculty
Charles University
Kateřinská 30
120 00 Prague 2, Czech Republic

Shunsuke Ohtahara, M.D.
Professor of Child Neurology
Department of Child Neurology
Okayama University Medical School
5-1, Shikatacho - 2 chome
Okayama 700, Japan

Lorcan O'Tuama, M.D.
Division of Nuclear Medicine
Department of Radiology
Children's Hospital
Boston, Massachusettes 02115

Scott B. Perlman, M.D.
Associate Professor
Department of Radiology
University of Wisconsin Hospital and
   Clinics
600 Highland Avenue
Madison, Wisconsin 53792

Stefano Ricci, M.D.
Section of Neurophysiology
"Bambino Gesù" Children's Hospital
Piazza S. Onofrio, 4
00165 Rome, Italy

Brian Robinson, M.D.
Department of Genetics
The Hospital for Sick Children
555 University Avenue
Toronto, Ontario, M5G 1X8 Canada

Robert S. Rust, M.D.
Assistant Professor
Department of Pediatrics and Neurology
University of Wisconsin Hospital and
   Clinics
600 Highland Avenue
Madison, Wisconsin 53792

Norio Sakuragawa, M.D.
Director
Department of Inherited Metabolic
   Diseases
National Institute of Neuroscience, NCNP
4-1-1, Ogawahigashi-cho
Kodaira, Tokyo, 187 Japan

Charles Scriver, M.D.

Professor of Pediatrics
McGill University
Montreal Children's Hospital
2300 Tupper Street
Montreal, Quebec, H3H 1P3 Canada

Hartmut Siemes, M.D.

Department of Pediatrics
Rittberg-Krankenhaus
Berlin, D-12205 Germany

Kenneth Silver, M.D., MSc.

Associate Professor of Pediatrics,
* Neurology and Neurosurgery*
Departments of Neurology, Neurosurgery,
* and Pediatrics*
McGill University
Montreal Children's Hospital
Montreal, Quebec, H3H 1P3 Canada

John C. Steele, M.D., F.R.C.P.(C)

Professor of Medicine
Department of Medicine
John A. Burns School of Medicine,
* Hawaii*
HCR 18 one 18
Umatac Village, Guam 96918

Donatella Tampieri, M.D.

Associate Professor of Radiology
Department of Radiology
Montreal Neurological Hospital and
* Institute*
McGill University
3801 University Street
Montreal, Quebec, H3A 2B4 Canada

Federico Vigevano, M.D.

Professor and Head
Section of Neurophysiology
Department of Paediatric Neurology
"Bambino Gesù" Children's Hospital
Piazza S. Onofrio, 4
00165 Rome, Italy

John Wilson, M.B., B.S., B.Sc.,
Ph.D., F.R.C.P

Consultant Neurologist
Department of Neurology
Great Ormond Street Hospital for
* Children*
Great Ormond Street
London, WC1N 3JH England

Benjamin G. Zifkin, M.D., C.M.,
F.R.C.P.(C)

Department of Neurological Sciences
Hôpital du Sacré-Coeur de Montreal
Epilepsy Clinic
Montreal Neurological Hospital and
* Institute*
3801 University Street
Montreal, Quebec, H3A 2B4 Canada

Emanuele Zullini, M.D.

Cattedra di Neuropsichiatria Infantile
Policlinico Borgo Roma
37134 Verona, Italy

Mary L. Zupanc, M.D.

Associate Professor of Child Neurology
Department of Child Neurology
Mayo Clinic
200 SW First Avenue
Rochester, Minnesota 55905

Series Foreword

The publication of *Alternating Hemiplegia of Childhood* in the International Review of Child Neurology Series fulfills the criteria that the International Child Neurology Association should improve the quality of care of children with neurological disorders. Each series volume is devoted to an in-depth examination of a particular topic, and this volume achieves that aim by examining this relatively unusual condition.

The International Child Neurology Association was founded in 1973 and has brought together child neurologists from all over the world who are dedicated to promoting clinical excellence and scientific research in child neurology. We are sure that this volume will be another step forward in achieving this aim.

Peter G. Procopis

Foreword

The golden years of clinical neurology, which began in the middle of the nineteenth century, practically drew to a close a century later, when most neurological syndromes had been recognized and appropriately classified. In the last 40 years, neurologists have had access to a wide range of diagnostic techniques. On the one hand, these have rendered the approach to the patient far more rewarding, allowing us to promptly confirm an anatomical lesion that could be only suspected on clinical grounds. On the other hand, the vast amount of information that can now be collected by these investigations appears to have relegated the traditional instruments of the clinician (a pen for writing the history and a hammer for examining the patient) to remnants of the dinosaur age. Yet this is only apparently so.

To begin with, the most sophisticated recent techniques have generally confirmed the diagnostic acumen of our forebears. A good example is found in the differences that molecular geneticists are now demonstrating among subtypes of neurodegenerative disorders, differences that match those of the clinical descriptions. Besides, there is still a place for clinical recognition of new syndromes. Alternating hemiplegia of childhood (AHC) is a typical example of a recently identified condition that is still in search of its etiology, its laboratory markers, and its effective therapy. The diagnosis of AHC still rests on the description that an astute historian can obtain from the anxious relatives, and on the information that the eye of the neurologist (admittedly with the aid of a video camera) can extract from these children's fussy, episodic behavior.

AHC teaches us other lessons, namely that the solution of the puzzle can come only from the joint efforts of neuroscientists of different backgrounds, in this case clinicians, geneticists, electrophysiologists, and functional neuroradiologists. We eagerly await a neurophysiological study of brainstem responses during an ophthalmoplegic spell, as well as functional magnetic resonance imaging during an episode of shifting hemiplegia. We also await a drug which, acting on an as yet unidentified neurotransmitter system, will stop the inexorable course of this condition. This book represents the results of a meeting in Rome which assembled the majority of neurologists and neuroscientists who have studied AHC. Each article is the sum of their experiences and the product of the fruitful discussions which followed their presentations. I believe this book provides a complete overview of the current knowledge of the syndrome, and as president of FOREP (Epilepsy and Related Syndromes Research Foundation), which sponsored the meeting, I am proud to introduce it. We hope that, with the hospitality of the "Bambino Gesù" Children's

Hospital and the organizational skills of Federico Vigevano, we can meet again soon for the purpose of writing the next chapter, this time on the prevention and cure of AHC.

Mario Manfredi
Professor of Neurology
Department of Neurological Sciences
University of Rome "La Sapienza"
Rome, Italy

Preface

The three editors of this volume share an abiding interest in alternating hemiplegia of childhood (AHC). The earliest description by Verret and Steele overlapped with accounts of more clearcut, classical migraine in childhood. Jean Aicardi first realized that AHC was an entity separate from migraine. As may be expected, the diagnosis still depends mainly on awareness of the syndrome. The causes of AHC have provoked many discussions among the three editors over the years. The relationship between AHC and migraine continues to be debated to this day. The ambiguity of this question was best described by Dr. John Wilson, who continues to be alternately attracted and repulsed by the migraine hypothesis.

Federico Vigevano and his colleagues investigated their young patients in depth. Intrigued by the mysterious nature of the disorder, they perceived the need to bring together and synthesize available information in order to establish a base for further research and progress. This was accomplished with the help of Professor Manfredi, the President of FOREP.

This monograph has resulted from the cooperation of many people who have had an interest in this intriguing disorder. It represents more than the sum of its parts: it leads to identification of a sui generis negative motor phenomenon, the alternating or unilateral hemiplegia which may occur as the signature of several childhood disorders, of which the classical form of AHC is the most common. Nowhere else have all the various disorders which manifest with this type of paralysis been examined critically, side-by-side.

Dr. Graham Lees, formerly of Raven Press, provided encouragement and guided the project through negotiations with the publisher. Judy Hummel and Mark Placito helped develop the book to its present format with patience, tact, and excellent judgment. We are grateful to Faye Rourke-Frew and Roula Vrentzos for their help with the manuscripts.

The editors of the ICNA series, Peter Procopis and Isabel Rapin recognized the utility of such a synthesis and deemed it worth presenting as a monograph.

There are almost as many contributors to this volume as there are patients, a tribute to the farsightedness of the series editors who agreed that even rare disorders deserve optimal scrutiny: certainly the parents of affected children have been grateful for the concern and the efforts of all contributors who tried to clarify the mechanisms of this dreadful disorder. Hopefully, their cooperation will provide both a basis and a stimulus for future research, improved understanding, and eventually, successful treatment and prevention.

Frederick Andermann
Jean Aicardi
Federico Vigevano

Alternating Hemiplegia of Childhood: A Historical Introduction and an Account of the Earliest Observations

John C. Steele

John A. Burns School of Medicine, Hawaii

In the late 1960s, soon after beginning work at The Hospital for Sick Children in Toronto as a pediatric neurologist, I cared for a child, Gerald M., who was about a year old. His unusual symptoms provoked my curiosity and he became the index case of the report on alternating hemiplegia of childhood.

Gerald was having attacks and his pediatrician asked my opinion about them. The situation was unclear in the beginning; just that he was having attacks during which he would get weak, and the weakness would be more on one side than the other. I interviewed Gerald's mother about his attacks and learned that when he was frustrated or angry, he would cry and seem to be in pain, clutch at his head, and soon after become weak and even paralyzed on one side or the other. Sometimes, he would be so weak on both sides that he couldn't move his arms or legs at all.

These were remarkable symptoms and I was not familiar with anything like them. Yet the history seemed quite definite and I was fortunate to witness an attack while he was admitted. As his mother had described, he was at first very fussy and irritable, and he repeatedly clutched at his head. He then became weak on one side and collapsed on his bed. Flaccid hemiparesis was profound, so that he had little movement of the arm or leg.

When I spoke with his mother and asked her about herself and her other children, she told me that for many years she had had headaches; sometimes they were just on one side, suggesting that they were vascular. She also mentioned that she had had an episode of weakness of her right limbs in association with a headache not long before. So it seemed to me, on the basis of her history and of Gerald's attacks, that it was possible that he was suffering from hemiplegic migraine and that his attacks of weakness were related to cerebral ischemia in association with migraine. What was so unique and astonishing was the very early age of onset. By his mother's account, the attacks had begun when he was only three months of age. He had an appropriate investigation to rule out a seizure disorder, and this included repeated and serial EEGs. He had a pneumoencephalogram and an arteriogram to exclude a tumor and/or vascular malformation; the latter was done soon after an attack to see if we could demonstrate any evidence of spasm. All the investigations were normal.

During the next several years, Gerald was repeatedly admitted to the hospital because of his attacks. His mother was distressed by them and kept bringing him back. We tried a host of medications including vasoactive drugs, anticonvulsants, and sedatives. None had any effect and his attacks remained frequent and impossible to control. Usually they lasted only a few hours, though on occasion he would remain paralyzed for days. As I followed him along during his admissions and as an outpatient, it became clear that his development was delayed. He was a slow and irritable child. Between his attacks, his neurological examinations were normal and he did not show any fixed deficit. I don't recall any involuntary movements. It was difficult to know whether his mild retardation was related to his recurrent and frequent spells, or whether it was inherited genetically.

I asked my neurological colleagues if they had met with patients like Gerald and whether AHC and childhood migraine were familiar to them. They had seen many children with paroxysmal disorders, and had attributed most of those to seizures. But Dr. Stobo Prichard, my Chief, and Dr. Doug McGreal recalled some children they had seen with alternating episodes of hemiplegia without convulsions.

When Dr. Simon Verret came to join me for six months as a resident from Dr. J. Clifford Richardson's Neurology training program at Toronto General Hospital, I encouraged him to search for other children with the same syndrome. With assistance from our Medical Records department and with help from Drs. Prichard and McGreal he was able to identify seven other young patients with alternating hemiplegia. In some of them, the symptoms had begun in the first year of life. Simon had them come to the hospital so we could reexamine them and review their interval histories. Most were much older by then and several were adolescents. Some were retarded. Some had dystonia and extrapyramidal movement disorders associated with their attacks but alternating hemiplegia was the hallmark. Unfortunately, I did not keep their records, so it has not been possible to review the group of patients again, and to follow up our initial report of 1971 (1).

My mentors in neurology were J. Clifford Richardson and Jerzy Olszewski. From Richardson, I learned to be observant and from Olszewski, to be curious. In 1964, our description of progressive supranuclear palsy (PSP) stemmed from Dr. Richardson's observations of a single patient in the 1950s (2). My original description of AHC with Verret also began with observations about an individual's illness. Throughout my medical career, I have focused on the individual and the anecdote because they delight me and they have scientific value. My studies of PSP with Richardson and Olszewski, multiple cranial nerve palsies with Aramsi Vasuvat (3), Mycoplasma pneumoniae infections with Richard Gladstone (4,5), migraine with Vladimir Hachinski and Peter Watson (6,7), fish poisoning (8) and now the amyotrophic lateral sclerosis/Parkinson-dementia complex of Guam with Tomasa Guzman (9), have all begun with curiosity about a patient who was unusual in some respect.

In this statistical era, it is imperative that individual observations and anecdotal accounts continue to be valued and encouraged. They are just as important as the statistically significant result. I am distressed when people are distrustful of anecdotal accounts and dismiss them in arbitrary fashion unless they are statistically validated. In the instance of AHC, I began the observation in one individual and then enlarged it by adding seven more. Other investigators went on to expand our initial observation, and the number of cases mounted. Now, through the efforts of Professors Frederick Andermann, Jean Aicardi, Federico Vigevano, and others, the number of patients with Alternating Hemiplegia of Childhood is sufficient to statistically validate descriptions of this condition. This was not possible when we first began.

The relationship between AHC and migraine is still being debated, but there will be a time when the mechanism of the attacks and the evolving neurological symptoms will be clarified, and Gerald M's illness will finally be understood. I am pleased to have begun this enquiry and I salute the many fine scientists who pursue it.

REFERENCES

1. Verret S, Steele JC. Alternating hemiplegia in childhood: A report of eight patients with complicated migraine beginning in infancy. *Pediatrics* 1971;47:675–680.
2. Steele JC, Richardson JC, Olszewski J. Progressive supranuclear palsy; A heterogeneous degeneration involving the brain stem, basal ganglia and cerebellum with vertical gaze and pseudobulbar palsy, nuchal dystonia and dementia. *Arch Neurol* 1964;10:333–359.
3. Steele JC, Vasuvat A. Recurrent multiple cranial nerve palsies: A distinctive syndrome of cranial polyneuropathy. *J Neurol Neurosurg Psychiat* 1970;33:828–832.
4. Steele JC, Gladstone RM, Thanasophon S, Fleming PC. Mycoplasma pneumoniae as a determinant of the Guillain-Barré syndrome. *Lancet* 1969;II:710–714.
5. Steele JC, Gladstone RM, Thanasophon S, Fleming PC. Acute cerebellar ataxia and concomitant infection with Mycoplasma pneumoniae. *J Pediatr* 1972;80:467–469.
6. Hachinski VC, Porchawka J, Steele JC. Visual symptoms in the migraine syndrome. *Neurology* 1973; 23:570–579.
7. Watson P, Steele JC. Paroxysmal dysequilibrium in the migraine syndrome of childhood. *Arch Otolaryngol* 1974;99:177–179.
8. Steele JC. Guam seaweed poisoning: Common marine toxins. *Micronesica* 1993;26:11–18.
9. Steele JC, Guzman T. Observations about amyotrophic lateral sclerosis and the parkinsonism-dementia complex of Guam with regard to epidemiology and etiology. *Can J Neurol Sci* 1987;14:358–362.

Clinical Delineation of the Syndrome

Alternating Hemiplegia of Childhood, edited by
Frederick Andermann, Jean Aicardi, and Federico Vigevano,
Raven Press, Ltd., New York © 1995.

1

Alternating Hemiplegia of Childhood: Clinical Findings and Diagnostic Criteria

Jean Aicardi, *Marie Bourgeois, and *Françoise Goutières

*Institute of Child Health, University of London, Mecklenburgh Square,
University of London, London WC1N 2AP, England; and *Department of Pediatrics,
Hôpital des Enfants Malades, 149 rue de Sèvres, 75743 Paris Cedex 15, France.*

The occurrence of transient attacks of hemiplegia involving alternatively either side of the body is an uncommon event in infants and children. Such attacks can result from a number of causes including hemiplegic migraine, vascular disorders, blood dyscrasias and, rarely, metabolic or demyelinating diseases. In such cases, hemiplegias are the only or predominant neurological manifestation and associated features are lacking or at least do not occur without hemiplegia being also present.

Alternating hemiplegia of childhood (AHC) was first reported in 1971 by Verret and Steele (1) who described three infants with typical features. However, these authors did not separate these three patients from five other children who appeared to present the classical picture of hemiplegic migraine of early onset. The latter patients did not exhibit the remarkable features of AHC that became clarified by later works. Two more cases that satisfied the description of AHC as currently understood were reported as basilar artery migraine by Golden and French (2) in 1978 and by Hockaday in 1979 (3). Hosking et al. (4) reported on five patients, two of which were fully described, and regarded the condition as being a form of complicated migraine. They did recognize some of the unusual features of their patients including the presence of mental retardation. Dittrich et al. in 1979 (5) gave a detailed description of the ocular and dystonic features in three patients and emphasized some of the remarkable clinical manifestations of the disorder. Krägeloh and Aicardi (6) gave a detailed account of the clinical symptoms and signs in five patients. They proposed that AHC was different from hemiplegic migraine and represented a specific severe disease with a poor neurological and mental outcome.

Approximately 75 cases have been reported so far (1–25). The characteristics of the condition have been outlined in several articles (7–9,18,25) and its possible relationship to migraine and epilepsy has been discussed (7,14,22).

In this chapter, we report 22 cases of AHC observed over a 24-year period at the Hôpital Saint Vincent de Paul and Hôpital des Enfants Malades, Paris (26), and review the literature on previously published cases. All our patients had repeated attacks of hemiplegia or hemiparesis that were associated in every case with other paroxysmal manifestations including dystonic attacks, episodes of paroxysmal nystagmus or abnormal eye movements, and autonomic disturbances. In all fully documented patients, episodes of bilateral hemiplegia occurred and going to sleep was always associated with a disappearance of the symptoms. The clinical picture was remarkably consistent as shown in Table 1. All children were personally examined by the senior author. The average duration of the disease before the most recent examination was 7 years 4 months (range 2 to 19 years, median 6.9 years).

In addition to clinical examination, all patients had one or several EEG tracings, 18 of which recorded clinically documented attacks. Eighteen had an enhanced CT scan and 11, a magnetic resonance scan. Results of special investigations that included angiography in nine patients, single photon emission computed tomography using [133]Xenon flow studies in four children, and pulsed Doppler study of carotid artery blood flow in four, are reported below. Sixteen patients underwent extensive biochemical studies including amino acid and organic acid studies, lactate determinations in blood and/or CSF, and endorphin level in CSF in 5 patients. Three patients had a muscle biopsy because of marked hypotonia in the first 3 months of life before they were seen at our institution.

CLINICAL FINDINGS

There were 12 girls and 10 boys aged 3 weeks to 11 months at the time of first examination. None had a family history of a similar disorder. In only three children was a family history of migraine or epilepsy in first- or second-degree relatives elicited, even though a systematic search for such antecedents was performed in all cases seen after 1980. Four patients were only children and most of the remaining were first or second children.

A history of abnormal pregnancy or delivery was present in only one twin, whose co-twin had been selectively aborted because of a neural tube defect. Three mothers had noted that fetal movements were weak, as compared with previous pregnancies.

Neurological abnormalities during the neonatal period had been noted in 10 infants. Seven were hypotonic, three were hyperexcitable, and five had difficulty in sucking or swallowing. For two children, the parents observed that the legs and/or arms momentarily turned purple without apparent reason and without obvious change in skin temperature. Four infants had a history of "convulsions" during the neonatal period but the exact nature of these episodes was difficult to define retrospectively. Jerking was not a prominent feature and it could well be that these events actually represented the first dystonic or ocular attacks. Indeed, abnormal eye movements were reported early by the parents of five infants. Interictal EEGs were normal but no record was obtained during an attack. Four children were given phenobarbital and two of them had no further episodes in the neonatal period. Two patients received assisted ventilation for periods of 24 to 48 hours because of apneic episodes that again might have been autonomic attacks of AHC.

TABLE 1. *Clinical features of individual patients*

Patient no.	Sex	Age and type of first attack	Age at first hemiplegia (mo)	Side predominance of hemiplegia	Epileptic seizures (age)	Severity of mental retardation	Severity of motor involvement	Age at end of follow-up
1	F	4 mo T/D+H	4	L	—	Severe	Severe	11 yr 6 mo
2	M	3 mo T/D	7	—	—	Severe	Severe	19 yr 6 mo
3	F	21 days T/D	6	L	—	Severe	Severe	4 yr 6 mo
4	M	6 mo H	6	—	—	Moderate	Moderate	11 yr
5	F	6 mo T/D+H	6	L	—	Severe	Moderate	7 yr
6	F	4 mo T/D	6	L	3, 7, 9 y	Severe	Moderate	16 yr
7	M	3 mo H	3	R	—	Mild	Mild	13 yr
8	M	2 mo N	8	R	—	Severe	Moderate	11 yr 1 mo
9	M	5 mo T/D+H	5	—	—	Borderline	Mild	11 yr 6 mo
10	F	3 mo T/D+H	3	L	—	Mild	Mild	9 yr 1 mo
11	F	11 mo H	11	—	11 y	Severe	Moderate	11 yr
12	M	4 mo N	5	L	—	Severe	Severe	5 yr 3 mo
13	M	5 mo R	10	R	3 yr 6 mo	Moderate	Moderate	6 yr
14	F	3 mo T/D	7	—	—	Mild	Moderate	7 yr
15	F	3 mo H	3	—	4, 5, 6 yr	Severe	Severe	7 yr 8 mo
16	F	21 days T/D	13	L	—	Borderline	Mild	6 yr 4 mo
17	M	2 mo T/D	4	L	2, 2½ y	Moderate	Moderate	2 yr 4 mo
18	M	20 mo N	8	R	—	Moderate or severe	Moderate or severe	4 yr
19	F	4 mo R	6	L	2 yr	?	Moderate	3½ yr
20	F	3 mo T/D	8	R	—	?	Moderate or severe	3 yr 7 mo
21	F	2 mo T/D	6	L	—	?	Moderate or severe	3 yr
22	M	4 mo T/D	5	L	—	?	Moderate	2 yr

T/D, tonic/dystonic; H, hemiplegia; N, nystagmus; R, respiratory disturbances.

Paroxysmal Manifestations

The first manifestations clearly related to AHC appeared in all patients before age 6 months and in six before age 3 months. Except for hypotonia that was present from birth in seven infants and for occasional feeding difficulties, they were *paroxysmal manifestations* that could appear as early as 10 days of age. Hemiplegia was not a feature at this early stage and only four infants had hemiplegia at the first attack, always in association with other paroxysmal symptoms. The most frequent early clinical manifestations at this stage were tonic or dystonic attacks and paroxysmal nystagmus.

Tonic or dystonic attacks were usually the earliest feature and were observed before 4 months of age in all but one infant. They were often unilateral with extreme stiffening of one side of the body, extension of ipsilateral limbs, and head turning toward the affected side with deviation of gaze in the same direction. Tonic contracture was often extreme, sometimes resulting in a rapid vibratory tremor. Most infants turned pale during attacks and they seemed to be in severe pain. Bilateral tonic attacks were less common but seemed quite painful with arching of the back, upward deviation of gaze, and intense crying. The mouth was tightly closed although drooling could occur. Sometimes there was lateral flexion of the trunk at the same time as opisthotonus.

In some infants, a unilateral attack could extend to involve secondarily the opposite side. The duration of tonic attacks rarely exceeded a few minutes. They occasionally recurred briefly during the following hours. Although they were initially the sole manifestation of an attack, up to the age of 13 months in one infant, they tended to be followed by hemiplegia during the second semester. The hemiplegias were regularly regarded as Todd's paralysis as they occurred following a tonic attack and were of brief duration. In several infants, the vibratory tremor that accompanied a tonic event, was interpreted as clonic jerking.

Tonic attacks were often associated with other paroxysmal manifestations even before the appearance of hemiplegias. These included paroxysmal nystagmus, autonomic changes, and paroxysmal dyspnea.

Paroxysmal nystagmus occurred in 18 of the 20 children for whom details were available. It was monocular in 14 cases and this was directly observed in several patients. The nystagmus was mainly horizontal in 13 and vertical in 3 cases. It was of large amplitude and appeared to be pendular in most of them but no oculographic recordings were performed. The nystagmus could switch from side to side in different attacks. The side involved was usually the same as that of the tonic and/or hemiplegic attacks, if any. Similarly the nystagmus could change from horizontal to vertical or vice versa in successive episodes. A few parents mentioned that there could be nystagmus in one eye and mydriasis in the other in some attacks. Episodes of isolated nystagmus were observed in 10 children. It was an early (probably even neonatal) manifestation. Most attacks lasted 30 seconds to 3 minutes, but in one child, bilateral, large amplitude nystagmus was almost permanent during bad periods. Paroxysmal strabismus occurred in nine children. In at least one infant for whom an ictal videotape was available, it presented as transient unilateral internuclear ophthalmoplegia, with absent adduction of the eye opposite the hemiplegia and limitation of abduction with nystagmus of the ipsilateral eye.

Paroxysmal autonomic phenomena were also early symptoms and could precede other manifestations of an attack or occur in isolation. The most common were paroxysmal dyspnea (see below) and vasomotor changes that included blanching or flushing of one limb or of half the body, with cold, clammy skin localized to one limb. These were usually seen on the same side as the hemiplegia that they regularly heralded in some cases.

Some children became hypothermic or hyperthermic during the acute episodes. Many appeared sleepy and yawned repeatedly but seemed to have difficulty falling asleep. Vomiting was only exceptionally observed and was never prominent.

Hemiplegic attacks were initially absent, brief, or inconspicuous and only progressively became the preponderant paroxysmal phenomenon. Twenty-one patients had had at least one hemiplegic attack by one year of age and the remaining child had it at 13 months of age. Hemiplegias could begin abruptly or progress over several minutes. Remarkably, the intensity of the hemiplegia fluctuated considerably from one moment to the next, occasionally disappearing briefly. The child could suddenly catch an object, then drop it, his arm hanging down cold, purplish, sometimes shaking slightly if he tried to use it, or he would suddenly collapse to one side because of his weak leg only to be able to stand again in a few minutes. In the course of prolonged attacks, the degree of weakness appeared to vary constantly from one minute to the next. Brief episodes of dystonic posturing often alternated with flaccid weakness. Attempts at using the paralyzed arm often resulted in tremor and/or the assumption of dystonic postures. In most cases, the hemiplegia was flaccid in type and no pyramidal tract signs were found except in three patients. Consciousness was preserved during attacks but may have been slightly depressed in some children who appeared quite drowsy. Patients were able to follow visually but head movements were slow and they responded only sluggishly to stimuli. A majority were fretful and cried out as if in pain, especially at the onset of an episode.

The arm was usually more severely affected than the lower limb but in many attacks, leg weakness was sufficiently marked to prevent walking or standing. The face was often spared or only minimally involved but marked facial weakness was seen in a few cases.

In all patients, both sides were involved but in 11 infants the hemiplegias were more frequent on the left side, in five on the right side, while there was an approximately equal distribution in six children. In cases with more frequent attacks on one side, the episodes tended to be more severe and to recover more slowly when the preferred side was involved. In some cases, only attacks starting on the preferred side became bilateral. Five children had a disturbance of speech, probably due to motor difficulties, in some attacks, regardless of the side involved.

The hemiplegias could shift from one side to the opposite during the same episode. Usually, there was a period of bilateral weakness when the second side became involved but in some patients, the change of side was abrupt, without bilateral paralysis.

Episodes of bilateral weakness occurred in all 20 patients for whom a complete history was available. They could occur suddenly or be heralded by a period of agitation, fatigue, and fretfulness lasting hours or days. Double hemiplegia usually occurred between 6 months and 2 years of age. Two types of bilateral attacks were recognized which could both occur in the same patient.

In 19 patients, bilateral movement was seen at the time hemiplegia was shifting from one side to the opposite. Bilateral weakness could last from an hour to more than a day and was associated with marked neurological deterioration. Fretfulness and apparent pain were considerably more intense than during unilateral attacks. Swallowing difficulties, drooling, slurred or indistinct speech, and choking on food or fluids were pronounced in 14 children and only mild in 5. Facial movements were also limited and the neurological picture was that of pseudobulbar involvement.

In 11 children, bilateral involvement was apparent from the start and did not follow a hemiplegic episode. Such attacks were marked by extreme hypotonia of the whole body with inability to move, while the level of consciousness was markedly depressed. The infants appeared to be in considerable distress. They could still follow visually but their response to stimuli was weak. Hypotonia was intermittently replaced by paroxysms of extreme stiffness with opisthotonic posturing lasting seconds to minutes. During prolonged bilateral episodes, waves of transient improvement alternated with periods of worsening with attenuated awareness, moaning, and fussiness. This second type of bilateral attack was often of great severity. At the end of an episode, the patients appeared exhausted and severe regression of their motor and cognitive abilities was common and could last several weeks. Indeed, loss of acquired skills such as walking, was apparently permanent in two infants following such severe attacks.

Some such episodes were associated with paroxysmal dyspnea in nine patients. However, dyspneic episodes also occurred in isolation in six children. Various respiratory abnormalities could be observed including shallow and slow breathing, expiratory difficulties with wheezing and episodes of polypnea. Such dyspneic episodes were usually mild but in at least one child, apneic episodes were responsible for a frightening deep cyanosis that appeared life-threatening. Vasomotor and ocular motor disturbances were also a frequent accompaniment of bilateral episodes.

The effect of sleep on the paralysis was remarkable and constant. All parents volunteered that resumption of symmetric movements followed immediately upon the child falling asleep. In prolonged attacks, paralysis in the same location reappeared 10 to 20 minutes after awakening. Even a short nap could result in brief remission of the paralysis, not necessarily associated with arrest of an attack. The end of a long-lasting episode was usually progressive over a few days but could be abrupt. Sleep has the same effect on bilateral attacks as on hemiplegias. Several parents took advantage of the brief period of normality following awakening to feed their child without the risk of choking and aspirating.

The frequency and duration of hemiplegias varied widely. The average interval between attacks was 24 to 48 hours in two patients, 48 hours to a week in eleven patients, 10 to 15 days in seven patients, and one month in two children. Brief episodes lasted from a few minutes to about an hour. Long attacks could last from several hours to several days, up to 2 weeks, with an average duration of 8 days. The total awake time with paralysis varied from a few hours monthly to up to 50% of total awake time in the most severely affected children. With increasing age, hemiplegic episodes followed a general pattern of initially increasing frequency and duration, followed by a plateau, then a decrease in the number and duration of attacks. However, hemiplegic episodes persisted at the end of follow-up in all cases including a patient observed for 19 years. In general, the paroxysmal manifestations associated with the hemiplegias, especially dystonic attacks and ocular abnormalities tended to decrease in frequency and intensity with time and usually disappeared after 5 to 7 years. At that point, the clinical picture was one of recurring pure hemiplegias, in sharp contrast to the picture of mainly dystonic, autonomic, and ocular symptoms observed in early infancy.

Precipitating factors seemed to exist in all children. Most commonly reported were emotional triggers and fatigue. Attacks were commonly precipitated by medical examination or by excitement such as often occurred at Christmas or at the time of birthday celebrations. Unusually hot or cold weather was held responsible by several parents and hot baths apparently induced episodes in five children. Bright lights were probably responsible for the frequent occurrence of attacks in supermarkets. In some children, the imminence of an attack was indicated by a change in behavior with aggressiveness, poor sleep, and sometimes speech difficulty and dribbling. In general, precipitating factors seemed to be more important in triggering hemiplegic attacks rather than episodes bilateral from the start.

Epileptic seizures were reported in six patients. One was recorded on video-tape by the parents and could be studied in some detail although no simultaneous EEG was available. The diagnosis of epilepsy was based on a clear description by parents of clonic jerking with or without loss of consciousness. The one seizure recorded on tape was unilateral, purely clonic, lasted more than 10 minutes, and occurred in full consciousness. Onset of the seizure was at the peak of an ipsilateral hemiplegic episode that had lasted for at least 20 minutes before the jerking began. In two other patients, seizures occurred at the peak of a bilateral episode while in the three remaining children they seemed independent of the hemiplegic attacks.

Nonparoxysmal Features

Marked hypotonia was present in all children and had probably existed from the first weeks of life. Results of muscle biopsy performed elsewhere were reported as normal.

Delay in passing motor milestones was common. Nine children had clearly abnormal motor development before onset of attacks. Head control was acquired between 5 and 15 months of age, sitting unsupported between one and 2 years, and bimanual coordination after one year of age. The other children seemed to develop reasonably well during the first year of life only to become retarded later. Independent walking was acquired by an average age of 42 months (range 23 months to 6 years) in 19 children and three patients, aged 3 years and 10 months to 5 years do not yet walk independently. Two patients have lost walking ability at 4 years and 7.5 years, respectively, following severe bilateral attacks. Fine motor control remained poor in all cases. Clumsiness was obvious early and everyday life activities such as dressing, tying knots or using a fork or knife were impossible or very difficult. Most children could not ride a bicycle and were poor at physical exercises and games.

Delayed cognitive development or mental retardation was present in all patients. Five children were mildly delayed or of borderline intelligence and 13 had moderate to severe cognitive difficulties. Four patients who were too young for formal assessment seemed to be severely retarded. Two children of borderline intelligence attended a normal class with special individual support. Learning difficulties were more marked for reading and writing than for counting or drawing. Most patients had great difficulties of attention and concentration and their behavior tended to be difficult and erratic. Temper tantrums and aggressiveness were frequent and tended to become more severe just before hemiplegic episodes. Autistic-like features were often noted. Some patients avoided personal contact and displayed gaze-avoidance. Their vocabulary could be rich but sentence construction required great effort. Some children spent their time studying the calendar or learning TV programs without ever watching them. One boy would read for hours at a time and seemed to enjoy this greatly but he was unable to tell what he had read and his parents thought he did not grasp the meaning of reading material. A child with an IQ of 80 had severe autistic features that prevented school integration.

Choreoathetotic movements were present in all cases but their intensity was variable. Some children had continuous choreic and/or athetotic movements that interfered with any form of voluntary motor activity while others had only mild instability with infrequent choreic jerks. In 10 children, a dystonic component with assumption of abnormal postures and slow torsion movement was observed, and clearly predominated on one side in one child. Interestingly, interictal choreoathetotic features were not seen in young infants during the early period of the disease at a time when the acute episodes often featured paroxysmal dystonia, but progressively increased in intensity and became continuous during wakefulness. The onset of interictal abnormal movements was within 2 years of onset in seven children, between 2 and 3 years in ten, and after 3 years in five, the longest interval being 5 years. School-age children often required typewriters or computers equipped with finger-guides as handwriting was often impossible.

Ataxia was also present in all cases and was essentially static in type. It was sometimes difficult to demonstrate because of the interference by the abnormal movements which disturbed balance and voluntary movements. The result was a puppet-like gait, the knees being maintained in recurvatum to help stabilize the patient.

Laboratory examinations were essentially negative (Table 2). Neuroimaging

TABLE 2. *Laboratory findings*

CT scan	$n = 18$	Normal	$n = 12$
		Mild atrophy	$n = 6$
MRI	$n = 11$	Normal	$n = 11$
Angiography	$n = 9$	Normal	$n = 9$
Pulsed Doppler study	$n = 4$	Normal	$n = 3$
		Abnormal	$n = 1$
SPECT using [133]Xenon (postictal period)	$n = 4$	Normal	$n = 2$
		Reduced regional cerebral blood flow	$n = 2$
EEG			
Ictal	$n = 18$	Moderate slowing	$n = 11$
		Normal	$n = 7$
Interictal	$n = 22$	Normal	$n = 22$
Visual evoked potentials	$n = 14$	Normal	$n = 14$
Electroretinogram	$n = 6$	Normal	$n = 6$
BAER	$n = 3$	Normal	$n = 3$
Somatosensory evoked responses	$n = 2$	Normal	$n = 2$
Karyotype (standard techniques)	$n = 4$	Normal	$n = 4$
Lactate determinations in blood and/or CSF	$n = 16$	Normal	$n = 16$
Endorphin level in CSF	$n = 5$	Normal	$n = 5$

studies including MRI in 11 patients gave normal results except for an occasional instance of mild to moderate cerebral atrophy. Angiography was normal in the nine patients in whom it was performed. Pulsed Doppler study of the carotid artery contralateral to the hemiplegia showed increased flow velocity in one child and no difference between sides in three other patients. SPECT using [133]Xenon flow studies was normal in two children and showed a mild decrease of perfusion on the ipsilateral side in two others interictally. No ictal study could be obtained as the children fell asleep at the time of examination as a result of sedation and this was associated with immediate disappearance of hemiplegia; thus the results corresponded to an immediate post-ictal period. The EEG was normal in 16 patients including 18 tracings obtained during an attack. Moderate slowing was seen in six cases either on the side opposite the hemiplegia or bilaterally. No epileptiform transients were seen but no clearly epileptic seizure was recorded.

Multiple types of treatment were tried. *Flunarizine* (5 to 10 mg daily) was used in 17 children. In 13 of them, the attacks appeared to be briefer and less severe but their overall frequency was not greatly reduced. The magnitude of the therapeutic effect varied widely. In one child the total time with hemiplegia was dramatically curtailed from about 50% to only brief episodes lasting less than an hour. In most, improvement was less marked. Increasing the dose to more than 10 mg daily did not appear to increase efficacy. Interestingly, any therapeutic effect obtained was obvious in a few days even though flunarizine has a prolonged half-life (19 days) and a steady state could not have been reached. No extrapyramidal side-effect has been observed even after 8.5 years of treatment. Several parents thought that their children had become aggressive while on the drug. Diazepam and phenytoin appeared to be of some help in two patients, each in association with flunarizine but their effect was never dramatic.

REVIEW OF PREVIOUSLY PUBLISHED CASES

The main features of 75 reported cases are shown in Table 3. The clinical picture is remarkably stereotyped, especially the occurrence of episodes of bilateral weakness, ocular motor disturbances, and the effects of sleep. In only one case was the lack of effect of sleep clearly described (3). One patient had attacks regularly starting during sleep (25) but also presented atypical features such as normal mentality so that inclusion of this case may not be warranted. All other reported patients were retarded or of borderline intelligence. Onset of the disease was almost always in the first year of life. Three of the five familial cases reported by Mikati et al. (23) had their first attack in the second or third year of life and were unusually mild in their nonictal features, especially with respect to mentality; two of them were able to lead relatively independent lives as adults.

The occurrence of unilateral nystagmus is one of the most curious features of the condition (5,6,25) but other oculomotor abnormalities, especially paroxysmal strabismus are also commonly mentioned. Fusco et al. (see Chapter 3) demonstrated unilateral paralysis of adduction similar to that observed in one of our patients.

Epileptic seizures occurred in addition to hemiplegic attacks in half the patients. Seizures most often occurred relatively late in the course and were mostly infrequent although status epilepticus or frequent attacks were occasionally described (25). Dalla Bernardina et al. (7) recorded electroclinical seizures in one of a pair of concordant monozygotic twins. The EEG was typical of a localized epileptic discharge while the clinical expression was limited to eye deviation and loss of consciousness. It seems likely that some of the attacks described as epileptic were actually tonic or dystonic seizures but true epileptic attacks undoubtedly occur.

The effect of flunarizine, initially reported by Casaer and Azou (27) has been

TABLE 3. *Main features in 75 previously reported cases[a]*

Feature	Number affected[b]
Hemiplegia involving either side	75/75
Episodes of double hemiplegia/quadriplegia	43/46
Tonic/dystonic attacks	50/52
Oculomotor abnormalities (nystagmus/gaze deviation/strabismus)	48/49
Disappearance of symptoms with sleep	36/38
Mental retardation	63/64
Neurological deficits (choreoathetosis/dystonia)	49/54

[a]Excluding cases of Krägeloh and Aicardi (ref. 6), Aicardi (ref. 8), and Casaer et al. (ref. 24).
[b]First figure indicates number of patients with this feature, second figure number of cases for which information was available.

confirmed in a controlled study of 12 patients by Casaer et al. (9) and, more recently by Silver and Andermann (25) in 10 children. Complete control of attacks is rare (9,25) and is probably only temporary. The main result of flunarizine therapy is a reduction in the duration and severity of the attacks rather than a reduction of their number. However, the effect is quite variable and 4 of the 10 patients of Silver and Andermann had no or only an insignificant reduction in attack duration. The frequency of hemiplegic attacks decreased moderately in only three of their patients (25).

Laboratory investigations in previously published cases have also been largely negative. Four patients underwent muscle biopsy specifically searching for evidence of mitochondrial disease and these biopsies were normal as was chromosome analysis in three cases (25). In the familial case of Makati et al. (23), a balanced reciprocal translocation 46 XY, t(3;9) (p26; q34) was found in the proband, in all the affected living relatives, and in one apparently unaffected sibling. Whether this chromosomal abnormality was etiologically related to the disease remains to be established. HMPAO-SPECT studies have given conflicting results (16,21–26; see also Chapter 5) with normal (25), decreased (15a; see also Chapter 5), or increased perfusion (21,22) of the contralateral hemisphere. Timing of the examination may be critical, with hypoperfusion at the onset of an attack followed by secondarily increased blood flow (21,24).

Other reported laboratory data include nuclear magnetic resonance spectroscopy of muscle in four patients, which showed a significant increase of inorganic phosphate (25) suggesting the possibility of widespread metabolic dysfunction.

Pathological data are scant. Bilateral hippocampal sclerosis was found in a 4-year-old patient but in three other cases no definite abnormalities were reported (25).

COMMENTS

The clinical features of AHC are remarkably similar with respect to both ictal and interictal phenomena. They include: 1) onset before 18 months of age; 2) repeated bouts of hemiplegia involving either side of the body at least in some attacks; 3) other paroxysmal disturbances including tonic/dystonic attacks, nystagmus, strabismus, dyspnea and other autonomic phenomena occurring during hemiplegic bouts or in isolation; 4) episodes of bilateral hemiplegia or quadriplegia starting either as generalization of a hemiplegic episode or bilateral from the start; 5) immediate disappearance of all symptoms on going to sleep, with recurrence 10 to 20 minutes after awakening in long-lasting bouts; 6) evidence of developmental delay, mental retardation and neurologic abnormalities including choreoathetosis, dystonia or ataxia. The most characteristic features are the occurrence of bilateral attacks that are not seen in any other neurologic disease of childhood, the presence of multiple paroxysmal manifestation, especially tonic attacks and oculomotor disturbances, and the consistent effect of sleep. Alternating episodes of hemiplegia on the other hand can be observed in many different disorders and have, in our experience, never been the only manifestation of AHC, especially during the first years of the course. Similarly, the age of onset can be slightly older in the mildest cases (23) and the nonparoxysmal features are nonspecific. These features cannot be considered as definite criteria for the disease as long as no biological marker is known. Their association, however, does not seem to occur in any other known condition and therefore allows a firm diagnosis to be made despite the lack of any characteristic laboratory abnormality. We believe that the few patients in which one or more essential features is lacking, such as absence of sleep effect and normal mentality in patient 8 of Silver and Andermann, should probably not be included until a laboratory marker is discovered.

One common cause of misdiagnosis is the failure to appreciate that AHC is a much more specific diagnosis than simply alternating or recurrent hemiplegia that can be observed in many different conditions (Table 4) and that hemiplegia need not be the most prominent clinical feature and may even be absent for several months at onset of the disorder.

Epilepsy is a very common misdiagnosis at an early stage. Lateralized tonic seizures, sometimes with vibratory tremor, followed by transient unilateral weakness are misinterpreted as seizures followed by Todd's paralysis. Moreover, true epileptic seizures may occur in patients with AHC. Ictal recordings remain normal or show only slowing during hemiplegic or dystonic attacks. (5–7). In some patients, interictal paroxysmal EEG abnormalities have been reported (22). On the whole AHC and epilepsy seem to be different conditions. The fact that epileptic seizures commonly occur at the peak of a hemiplegic attack (26) suggests that they may be a secondary phenomenon, perhaps related to local circulatory changes.

Hemiplegic migraine was not initially separated from AHC (1–4) and the recent international classification of headache has included AHC as a childhood periodic syndrome that may be associated with migraine (28). At variance with other investigators (1–4,25), we were not able to find an unusually high familial incidence of migraine in our cases. Furthermore, the onset of classic hemiplegic migraine is rarely before 2 years of age and the dystonic and ocular motor features are not reported. The EEG in hemiplegic migraine shows very marked, lateralized, slow wave activity that often persists for several days, or even weeks, postictally. The occurrence of mental retardation and/or neurologic sequelae is exceptional in migraine and generally results from strokes that are rare in children (29). Despite a somewhat similar effect of sleep and occasional reports of throbbing headache, nausea, paresthesia, photophobia, and phonophobia in patients with a clinical picture consistent with AHC (3,25; J. Stephenson, *personal communication*, 1991), AHC is too different from basilar or hemiplegic migraine to be regarded as being part of the migraine spectrum. Unusual syndromes have been related to migraine and may present with very severe and unusual clinical and EEG characteristics. These include a syndrome of familial cerebellar ataxia and continuous myokymia (30) and one of migraine, coma, visual hallucinations, and progressive cerebellar ataxia (31). We have observed a 13-year-old girl with repeated episodes of deep

TABLE 4. *Differential diagnosis of AHC*

Migraine and related conditions
  Hemiplegic migraine
  Basilar migraine
  Migraine, coma, and visual hallucinations
Vascular disorders
  Arteriovenous malformations
  Multiple emboli from cardiac sources, e.g., atrial myxomas
  Hereditary hemorrhagic telangiectasia (Osler-Weber-Rendu disease)
Blood coagulation or viscosity disturbances
  Homocystinuria
  Thrombocythemia
  Other coagulation disorders?
Epilepsy
  Inhibitory seizures
  Postictal (Todd's) hemiplegia
Metabolic diseases
  Mitochondrial disorders, especially mitochondrial encephalomyopathy with
    lactic acidosis and stroke-like episodes (MELAS)
  Leigh's subacute encephalomyelopathy
  Pyruvate dehydrogenase deficiency
  Ornithine transcarbamylase (heterozygous forms) and other ammonia cycle enzyme deficiencies
  Intermittent forms of amino acid and organic acid disorders
Others
  Paroxysmal dyskinesias
    Paroxysmal choreoathetosis (Mount and Reback)
    Atypical kinesigenic dyskinesias or dystonias
  Paroxysmal torticollis of infancy
  Paroxysmal cerebellar ataxia and myokymia
  Demyelinating diseases
    Multiple sclerosis
  Acute disseminated encephalomyelitis (prolonged forms)
  Schilder's disease

coma, sometimes with life-threatening respiratory problems requiring intubation, and with prolonged EEG changes amounting to almost flat tracings for several days. This patient had had typical episodes of migraine and recovered completely after each episode, some of them featuring hemiplegia.

The possibility that AHC may represent a type of mitochondrial disease is attractive, in view of the superficial resemblance of the condition to mitochondrial encephalomyopathy with lactic acidosis and stroke-like episodes (32,33). However, there is usually no vomiting in AHC, the episodes are more prolonged, and associated signs are different. Imaging techniques, especially MRI, show areas of altered signal or density (34) and the overall course is more severe than that of AHC, at least with respect to outlook for life and systemic disease. Atypical (35) or hitherto undescribed mitochondrial disorders cannot be excluded as a cause of AHC even though high lactate levels in blood and CSF have never been found and muscle biopsy specimens have not shown ragged-red fibers, or abnormalities of respiratory chain enzymes (25; M. L. Zupanc, *personal communication*, 1992) making this hypothesis unlikely.

Paroxysmal dyskinesias especially of the non-kinesigenic type (36) are not associated with paralysis, abnormal eye movements, or cognitive deterioration. At an early stage of AHC, however, the dystonic features may be so prominent that paroxysmal dyskinesias may be considered. Paroxysmal torticollis of infancy may pose a diagnostic problem because of similar age of onset, heat turning and tilting to one side, usually alternating in successive attacks, and especially because stiffness and dystonic posture may affect an entire side of the body, last several hours, and be associated with fussiness and apparent pain. However, there is usually no nystagmus and no associated features develop over time.

In several of our patients, the attacks were interpreted as malingering or "hysteria" because of the bizarre dystonic features during attacks, preserved awareness, and frequent triggering by psychological stimuli. The unusual behavioral features of these children and the fluctuation in intensity of the weakness that can disappear or reappear suddenly were regarded as supporting a "psychiatric" condition. The parents of one child were suspected of trying to fraudulently obtain welfare benefits because the child was examined outside an episode and the history appeared "suspicious."

Rare differential diagnoses are shown in Table 4. An occasional case of Osler-Weber-Rendu disease can present with alternating hemiplegia although without the distinctive features of AHC (37). Three patients with congenital cutis marmorata congenita presented with repeated transient episodes of alternating hemiplegia that would closely simulate AHC but the cutaneous abnormality was distinctive (38). Other vascular diseases are unlikely to produce repeated and typical episodes.

The etiology of AHC is unknown. No detectable morphologic anomalies of the brain have been found and no significant antecedent recorded. Most imaging studies have been normal and the only abnormality described is mild atrophy which is more likely a consequence rather than a cause of the disorder. The disease is usually sporadic and only one familial case affecting four (possibly five) patients in two generations is known (23). The disorder in this family was quite typical with unilateral and bilateral attacks, dystonia, ocular motor abnormalities, and disappearance of the symptoms with sleep. Onset was later than usual in two members and the oldest patients could live a relatively independent life as adults. These features, if confirmed, would suggest that familial cases may differ slightly from the usual sporadic cases.

The mechanisms responsible for the symptoms and signs of AHC are poorly understood. Vascular or circulatory disturbances affecting predominantly the vertebrobasilar circulation would account for alternating hemiplegias, movement disorders, and signs and symptoms of brainstem involvement such as nystagmus or internuclear ophthalmoplegia. They would not, however, satisfactorily explain the cognitive deficit. One of the major and unresolved issues is whether AHC is a static encephalopathy or a progressive condition and what role, if any, the repetition of acute attacks plays in the deterioration. Many infants with AHC have neurodevelopmental abnormalities very early in life and repeated assessment of cognitive abilities that would be necessary to demonstrate regression is not yet available. Clearly, severe bilateral attacks may be associated with neurological deterioration (e.g., loss of ability to walk or speak) which may take weeks to recover and may, in fact, leave permanent sequelae, with resulting stepwise deterioration. In some patients, initial development may be relatively normal with obvious deterioration only after 2–3 years of age.

In some cases, atrophy seems to appear on imaging after a few years but serial studies are not available. Some patients with severe neurodevelopmental abnormalities still have normal imaging studies after several years, although acquired microcephaly seems to be common. Other studies, such as evoked visual or somatosensory responses and repeated HMPAO-SPECT also suggest progressive impairment of CNS function (see Chapter 5) but still require confirmation. Our clinical impression is that the disorder may be progressive for the first 1 to 3 years, then stabilize at least with regard to mental status. There is no doubt, however, that the movement disorder is not present from onset but appears after one to several years and is progressive in the early stages of the disorder. The role of repeated attacks in aggravating of the disease is unclear. In some patients, severe neurodevelopmental impairment was observed despite suppression of acute attacks for periods of up to 2 years. Consequently, the value of flunarizine treatment in preventing deterioration remains unproven whereas its effect on the duration and severity of attacks is established (9,25).

REFERENCES

1. Verret S, Steele JC. Alternating hemiplegia in childhood: A report of eight patients with complicated migraine beginning in infancy. *Pediatrics* 1971;47:675–680.
2. Golden GS, French JH. Basilar artery migraine in young children. *Pediatrics* 1975;56:722–726.
3. Hockaday JM. Basilar artery migraine in childhood. *Dev Med Child Neurol* 1979;21:455–463.
4. Hosking GP, Cavanagh NPC, Wilson J. Alternating hemiplegia: complicated migraine of infancy. *Arch Dis Child* 1978;53:656–659.
5. Dittrich J, Havlóva M, Nevšímalová S. Paroxysmal hemiparesis of childhood. *Dev Med Child Neurol* 1979;21:800–807.
6. Krägeloh I, Aicardi J. Alternating hemiplegia in infants: Report of five cases. *Dev Med Child Neurol* 1980;22:784–791.
7. Dalla Bernardina B, Capovilla G, Trevisan E, et al. Alternating hemiplegia of infants. In: Andermann F, Lugaresi E, eds. *Migraine and epilepsy.* London: Butterworths; 1987;189–201.
8. Aicardi J. Alternating hemiplegia of childhood. *International Pediatrics* 1987;2:115–119.
9. Casaer P. Flunarizine in alternating hemiplegia in childhood. An international study of 12 children. *Neuropediatrics* 1987;18:191–195.
10. Robaszewska U. Diagnostic difficulties in paroxysmal alternating hemiplegia in a child. *Neurol Neurochir Pol* 1976;10:415–418.
11. Ritz A, Jacobi G, Emrich R. Komplizierte Migräne beim Kind. *Monatsschr Kinderheilkd* 1981; 129:504–512.
12. Curatolo P, Cusmai R. Drugs for alternating hemiplegic migraine [Letter]. *Lancet* 1984;2:980.
13. Tada H, Miyake S, Hayashi M, Iwamoto H. A pathophysiological study of alternating hemiplegia in childhood. *Brain Dev* 1985;7:2:207.
14. Andermann F, Silver K, Saint-Hilaire MH, et al. Paroxysmal alternating hemiplegia of childhood: Treatment with Flunarizine and other agents. *Neurology* 1986;36[Suppl 1]:327.
15. Sakuragawa N, Arima M, Matsumoto S. Nationwide investigation of alternating hemiplegia of children. *Journal of the Japan Pediatric Society* 1988;92:892–898.
15a. Sakuragawa N, Matsuo T, Kihira S, et al. Alternating hemiplegia in infancy: Two case reports and reduced regional cerebral blood flow in $^{11}CO_2$ dynamic position emission tomography. *Brain Dev* 1985;7(2):207.
16. Siemes H, Casaer P. Alternierende Hemiplegie des Kindesalters. Klinischer Bericht und SPECT-Studie. *Monatsschr Kinderheilkd* 1988;136:467–470.

17. Siemes H. Rectal chloral hydrate for alternating hemiplegia of childhood [Letter]. *Dev Med Child Neurol* 1990;32:931.
18. Campistol Plana J, San Fito A, Pineda Marfa M, Fernandez-Alvarez E. Hemiplegia alternante en la infancia: forma de presentacion, evolution y tratamiento en tres observaciones. *An Esp Pediatr* 1990;32(4):336–338.
19. Shirasaka Y, Ito M, Okuno T, Mikawa H, Yamori Y. Epileptic seizures difficult to differentiate from alternating hemiplegia in infants: A case report. *Brain Dev* 1990;12:521–524.
20. Santanelli P, Guerrini R, Dravet C, et al. Brainstem auditory evoked potentials in alternating hemiplegia: ictal vs interictal assessment in one case. *Clin Electroencephalogr* 1990;28:51–54.
21. Zupanc ML, Dobkin JA, Perlman SB. ^{123}I-iodoamphetamine SPECT brain imaging in alternating hemiplegia. *Pediatr Neurol* 1991;7:35–38.
22. Kanazawa O, Shirasaka Y, Hattori H, Okuno T, Mikawa H. Ictal ^{99m}Tc-HMPAO SPECT in alternating hemiplegia. *Pediatr Neurol* 1991;7:121–124.
23. Mikati MA, Maguire H, Barlow CF, et al. A syndrome of autosomal dominant alternating hemiplegia: clinical presentation mimicking intractable epilepsy; chromosomal studies; and physiologic investigations. *Neurology* 1992;42:2251–2257.
24. Aminian A, Strashun A, Rose A. Alternating hemiplegia of childhood: Studies of regional cerebral blood flow using ^{99m}Tc-hexamethyl-1 propylene amine oxime single-photon emission computed tomography. *Ann Neurol* 1993;33:43–47.
25. Silver K, Andermann F. Alternating hemiplegia of childhood: A study of 10 patients and results of Flunarizine treatment. *Neurology* 1993;43:36–41.
26. Bourgeois M, Aicardi J, Goutières, F. Alternating hemiplegia of childhood. *J Pediatr* 122:673–679.
27. Casaer P, Azou M. Flunarizine in alternating hemiplegia in childhood [Letter]. *Lancet* 1984;2:579.
28. Olesen J. Classification and diagnostic criteria for headache disorders. *Cephalalgia* 1988;8[Suppl 7]:26.
29. Rossi LN, Penzien JM, Deonna T, Goutières F, Vassella F. Does migraine related stroke occur in childhood? *Dev Med Child Neurol* 1990;32:1016–1021.
30. Brunt ERP, Van Weerden TW. Familial paroxysmal kinesigenic ataxia and continuous myokymia. *Brain* 1990;113:1361–1382.
31. Fitzsimons RB, Wolfenden WH. Migraine coma: meningitic migraine with cerebral oedema associated with a new form of autosomal dominant cerebellar ataxia. *Brain* 1985;108:555–577.
32. Pavlakis SG, Rowland LP, De Vivo DC, Bonilla E, Di Mauro S. Mitochondrial myopathies and encephalomyopathies. In: Plum F, ed. *Advances in contemporary neurology*. Philadelphia: FA Davis; 1988;95–123.
33. Montagna P, Galassi R, Medori R, et al. MELAS syndrome: characteristic migrainous and epileptic features and maternal transmission. *Neurology* 1988;30:751–754.
34. Matthews PM, Tampieri D, Berkovic SF, Andermann F, Silver K, Chitayat D, Arnold DL. Magnetic resonance imaging shows specific abnormalities in the MELAS syndrome. *Neurology* 1991;41:1043–1046.
35. Dvorkin GS, Andermann F, Carpenter S, et al. Classical migraine, intractable epilepsy and multiple strokes: a syndrome related to mitochondrial encephalomyopathy. In: Andermann F, Lugaresi E, eds. *Migraine and epilepsy*. London: Butterworths; 1987;203–232.
36. Bressman SB, Fahn S, Burke RE. Paroxysmal non kinesigenic dystonia. *Adv Neurol* 1988;80:403–413.
37. Myles ST, Needham CW, Leblanc FE. Alternating hemiplegia associated with hereditary hemorrhagic telangiectasia. *Can Med Assoc J* 1970;103:509–511.
38. Baxter P, Gardner-Medwin D, Green SH, Moss C. Congenital livedo reticularis and recurrent stroke-like episodes. *Dev Med Child Neurol* 1993;35:917–926.

Alternating Hemiplegia of Childhood, edited by
Frederick Andermann, Jean Aicardi, and Federico Vigevano,
Raven Press, Ltd., New York © 1995.

2

Alternating Hemiplegia of Childhood: The Natural History of the Disorder in a Group of 10 Patients

Kenneth Silver and Frederick Andermann

Montreal Children's Hospital, the Departments of Neurology, Neurosurgery, and Pediatrics, McGill University, Montreal Neurological Hospital and Institute, 3801 University Street, Montreal, Quebec H3A 2B4, Canada.

Alternating hemiplegia of childhood (AHC) is a rare syndrome characterized by frequent transient attacks of hemiplegia involving either side of the body.

The disorder is not widely known and only about 30 patients have been previously described in the literature (1–7). Onset is prior to 18 months of age with repeated attacks of hemiplegia involving either or both sides. Children usually have other paroxysmal disturbances including ocular motor and autonomic manifestations, as well as intermittent dystonic posturing and choreoathetosis. Cognitive and neurological deficits become progressively more apparent over the years.

In a typical attack, the infants have a prodrome of screaming, restlessness, and appear to be in pain. Ocular motor abnormalities appear early. Surprisingly there may be unilateral nystagmus but this may also be bilateral and episodes of dystonic stiffening frequently occur. In the early stages of the illness the children may be hypotonic between attacks. Some have normal development before the onset of hemiplegic episodes whereas others may be delayed from the onset. Subsequently, multiple attacks of flaccid hemiplegia develop lasting anywhere from minutes to days at a time. Paralysis is often accompanied by autonomic symptoms such as alterations in skin color, temperature, and sweating. The hemiplegia can have a sudden or gradual onset and even fluctuate during an attack (8). In some patients bilateral hemiplegic attacks occur, manifested by generalized flaccidity, often associated with bulbar features such as dysphagia, dysarthria, and respiratory difficulty. In the bilateral attacks the level of consciousness may be reduced but unconsciousness does not develop. The episodes are dramatically relieved by sleep but may recur after the child wakes. An association with migraine has been noted since the earliest description (1).

We had the opportunity to examine and follow 10 patients ranging in age up to 27

19

TABLE 1. *AHC: Clinical features in 10 patients*

Patient	1	2	3	4
Sex	F	F	F	M
Age (yr)	27	10	14	8
Symptoms onset (mo)	3	3	5	3
Hemiplegia onset (mo)	7	7	7	9
Frequency/mo	20	3	3	20
Duration (min/hr/days)	2 hr	6 hr	5 days	3 hr
Provoking trigger	Light, excitement	Light, excitement	Activity, foods	Excitement, bathing
Seizures	Status	Rare	0	0
Neurological exam	Microcephally, hypotonia, choreoathtosis	Hemiparesis, hypotonia, ataxia, tremor	Dysarthria, chorea, hypotonia, hyperactivity	Athetosis, dystonia
Developmental/cognitive delay	Severe	Mild	Moderate	Borderline

years (9). They had a mean age of 11.0 years and the youngest was 3 years old (Table 1). Mean age at onset of their first neurological symptoms was 3.8 months (range 3 to 6 months). Initially nystagmus or dystonia or both were seen in 6 of the 10 children (Fig. 1). Dystonic attacks consisted of generalized or focal stiffening sometimes with head deviation or turning lasting from a few minutes up to 1 hour. Several attacks could occur during the same day. Episodic nystagmus occurred either alone or together with the dystonic attacks. The nystagmus was usually monocular and in one child was associated with pupillary dilatation. Some of the other patients developed episodic screaming, tremor, obtundation, or breath holding spells prior to the onset of recurrent hemiplegia.

The diagnosis of alternating hemiplegia of childhood was made only after a mean interval of 4.8 years (range 2 to 18 years) from the onset of the first symptoms (Fig. 2). Hemiplegic attacks were first noted at a mean age of 9.0 months (range 7 to 13 months). In some, the hemiplegia was noted immediately after the cessation of recurrent paroxysmal dystonia. However, in most patients the dystonic attack and episodes of nystagmus diminished in frequency after the first year and the hemiplegic episodes became more prominent thereafter. The hemiplegia could develop suddenly or have a gradual onset over minutes. Hemiplegic attacks occurred at a mean frequency of 11 per month (range 2 to 20). Their duration fluctuated between patients, and varied also in the same patient; they lasted from minutes to 7 days. However, there was a tendency for the majority of attacks to last for a similar period in any given patient. In two children the attacks usually lasted for minutes, in four they lasted hours, and in four the duration was of the order of days (Fig. 3). In the habitual events there was marked flaccid paralysis of the arm with moderate weakness in the leg and milder facial involvement. Each episode reached a peak over a

TABLE 1. *Continued.*

5	6	7	8	9	10
M	F	F	M	F	F
9	8	17	3	4	10
6	3	5	4	3	3
13	NR	12	8	9	9
3	2	8	20	8	15
4 days	2 hr	days	20 min	5 hr	days
NR	Light, excitement	Noise, excitement	Sleep	Fatigue, excitement	None
0	Frequent	Rare	0	Rare	0
Athetosis, dystonia	Ataxia, hypotonia, choreoathetosis	Hyperreflexia, + Babinski	Normal	Hypotonia, in-toeing,	Ataxia, incoordination
Borderline	Mild	Mild	Normal	Borderline	NR

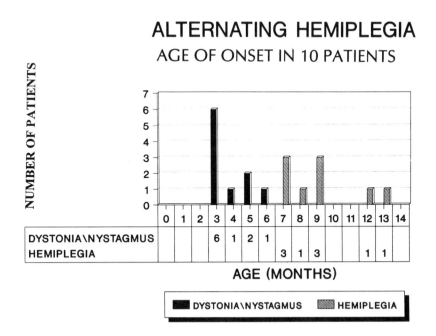

ALTERNATING HEMIPLEGIA
AGE OF ONSET IN 10 PATIENTS

NUMBER OF PATIENTS

	0	1	2	3	4	5	6	7	8	9	10	11	12	13	14
DYSTONIA\NYSTAGMUS				6	1	2	1								
HEMIPLEGIA								3	1	3			1	1	

AGE (MONTHS)

DYSTONIA\NYSTAGMUS   HEMIPLEGIA

FIG. 1. Distribution of patients according to the age of onset of neurological symptoms: dystonia and/or nystagmus and hemiplegic attacks. In one patient time of onset of hemiplegia was not documented.

ALTERNATING HEMIPLEGIA
AGE DISTRIBUTION (N=10)

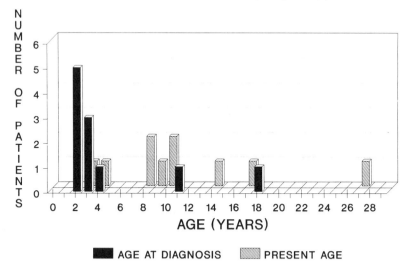

FIG. 2. Distribution of patients according to the age when AHC was diagnosed and their present age.

ALTERNATING HEMIPLEGIA (N=10)

FREQUENCY   DURATION

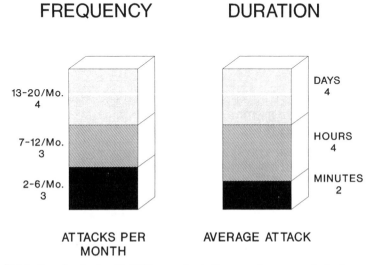

FIG. 3. Distribution of patients with AHC according to the mean frequency of attacks per month and mean duration of attacks.

few minutes; the degree of deficit varied from mild to severe paralysis. During the hemiplegic attacks consciousness and some speech were preserved.

Eight patients were found to have bilateral hemiplegic attacks. In one these occurred as often as 5 times per month and the duration was up to several days. Three patients averaged one bilateral episode per month and in four, bilateral events occurred only occasionally. During these bilateral attacks the patients were anarthric, dysphagic, and had a more severe flaccid or dystonic generalized paralysis. They were, however, conscious, able to comprehend, and follow verbal commands.

In four patients attacks occurred more often on the right side and in two on the left; no lateralization was noted in the remaining four. In six children pallor and coldness of the affected extremities were described and one had flushing of the face during attacks.

In seven patients exposure to bright light or excitement precipitated the episodes. Other provoking factors were bathing, loud noise, specific foods, or anticonvulsant medication such as primidone. In patient 8, attacks occurred exclusively out of sleep and he was the only one who showed this pattern. One and a half hours after falling asleep he would awaken with a scream, cry incessantly, and then develop hemiplegia. Attacks lasted for about 20 minutes: he would then return to sleep for the remainder of the night, awakening normal the following morning. In six other children the attacks would cease when they went to sleep or had a nap. Sleep could last for only a few minutes and they would awaken with the hemiplegia resolved.

Six of the eight pregnancies of the mothers were described as uneventful. Two mothers had increased migraine headaches while pregnant. There were no perinatal difficulties, but three infants were described to have seizures, apnea, or tremors though precise documentation of these complications was not available.

There was a prominent family history of migraine, mainly without aura, in six of the mothers and in three of the fathers. In some families other members also had migraine, usually common. There were no first or second degree family members with other neurological disorders, alternating hemiplegia or epilepsy.

Developmental milestones were globally delayed (Fig. 4). Affected children sat at a mean age of 9.3 months (range 8 to 14), walked at 25 months (range 16 to 72), said their first few words at 18 months (range 12 to 36) and sentences at 46.8 months (range 24 to 72). Patient 1 at age 27 years is still not able to communicate in sentences. Of the nine patients studied two had borderline cognitive function, four had mild retardation, one was moderately mentally retarded, and 1 had severe retardation. Patient 8, the boy with attacks arriving out of sleep is the only one with normal developmental neurological and cognitive status at 3 years of age.

Five of the ten patients had epileptic seizures in addition to their hemiplegic attacks. Patient 1 developed tonic-clonic seizures at 12 years of age; initially attacks were well controlled with valproic acid. In her mid twenties she had recurrent attacks of status epilepticus and a unilateral frontal focal epileptogenic EEG abnormality. Three patients had rare seizures (patients 2, 7, and 9) controlled by medication and patient 6 had several generalized tonic-clonic seizures per month.

Neurological examination between hemiplegic attacks showed abnormalities in

ALTERNATING HEMIPLEGIA
DEVELOPMENT (N=10)

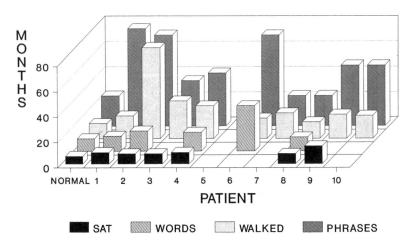

FIG. 4. Developmental milestones achieved by patients. Delays were more evident as the children grew older.

nine of the patients (Table 1). Hypotonia, ataxia, and choreoathetosis were frequent. Dystonia, spasticity, and microcephaly were seen less often.

Laboratory investigations did not reveal any specific abnormality (Table 2). All patients had CT Scans, eight had cerebral angiograms, six had MRI scans, and two had PET scans. Several of these investigations were repeated on more than one occasion in each patient and were normal. Three patients had a ^{99m}Tc-HMPAO SPECT scan. This revealed a normal study in one patient and a reduced unilateral temporal regional uptake interictally in another; a third patient had a normal SPECT scan during a hemiplegic attack.

All patients had multiple EEG recordings. Three had normal interictal tracings, five showed diffuse slowing and three had epileptiform abnormalities. EEGs recorded in four patients during an attack of hemiplegia showed contralateral slow waves without epileptiform discharges. Three patients had evoked potentials (ABR and SER) performed interictally and these were normal. Four patients had muscle or liver biopsies specifically searching for evidence of mitochondrial disturbance and no abnormalities were found. Chromosome analysis was normal in three.

Four patients underwent nuclear magnetic resonance spectroscopy (MRS) of muscle (patients 1, 2, 8, and 9) and there was significant increase of inorganic phosphate in all (see Chapter 11).

The natural history and long-term prognosis of alternating hemiplegia was difficult to evaluate. Hemiplegic attacks were more severe during the first decade; later

TABLE 2. *Results of investigations*

Normal				Abnormal	
CT	10/10			Interictal EEG	
Angiogram	8/8	Muscle biopsy	3/3	diffuse slow	5/10
MRI	6/6	Liver biopsy	1/1	epileptiform	2/10
PET	2/2	Evoked potentials	3/3	Ictal EEG	
				focal slow	3/4
SPECT	2/3	Biochemistry	9/9	SPECT	1/3
EEG	3/10	Karyotype	3/3	MRS of muscle	4/4

they tended to be milder, but never resolved spontaneously. The cognitive delay became more evident over time (Fig. 5).

These 10 children with alternating hemiplegia have had many attacks of transient weakness over several years. The initial symptoms of the syndrome followed a clear temporal pattern. Early hypotonia or nystagmus preceded the onset of hemiplegia, usually by several months. The early symptoms commonly resolved over time and frequent attacks of hemiplegia emerged as the predominant manifestation. The complexity and fluctuation of these symptoms, as well as the lack of awareness, accounted for the usual delay of several years before the correct diagnosis was made and for the initial misdiagnosis of epilepsy in most of these patients.

Development was initially mildly delayed and some children were hypotonic. As they grew older the developmental lag and retardation became more apparent. In none of 9 patients studied was there evidence for developmental regression but rather a pattern of failure to progress along previous developmental gradients emerged. We attempted to determine the outcome of the original patients reported by Verret and Steele 1971 (1) but their records could not be located.

From previous reports (1–5) and from our present study it was difficult to be certain if the psychomotor delay was due to the underlying process or to the frequent attacks of hemiplegia and dystonia themselves.

Although half the patients had associated epileptic seizures there was no evidence that the hemiplegic attacks themselves were epileptic (7). Video EEG telemetry recordings during these episodes showed no epileptogenic discharges. They did not represent unilateral atonic or inhibitory seizure nor were they suggestive of a postictal or Todd's paralysis. The hemiplegic attacks were also unresponsive to anticonvulsants.

Though a vascular etiology had been suspected early, neuroimaging and angiographic studies did not reveal any evidence of cerebral vascular disease. In particular conditions like arteriovenous malformations, moya-moya syndrome, and hereditary hemorrhagic telangiectasia have not been found (10).

Recent studies using SPECT scanning in patients with alternating hemiplegia (11–13) showed conflicting results: normal, hyper-, or hypoperfusion of the contralateral hemisphere was found during a hemiplegic attack.

Metabolic disorders such as mitochondrial cytopathies may produce reversible

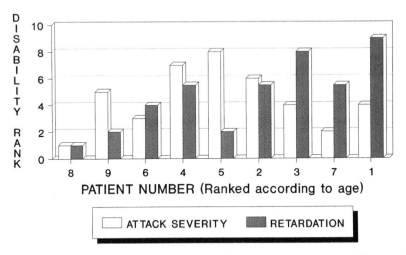

FIG. 5. Patients ranked according to age: no. 8 was the youngest and no. 1 the oldest (x-axis). The disability rank was the severity of hemiplegic attacks (duration times frequency per month) and the severity of mental retardation. The hemiplegic attacks worsened during the first decade, then improved. Intellectual deficit became more obvious in older patients.

focal neurological deficit including hemiplegia. None of our patients had the stroke-like lesions or basal ganglia calcifications seen in MELAS syndrome (14,15). No abnormalities of lactate, pyruvate, blood gases, or evidence of ragged red fibers were found (16,17). However NMR spectroscopic abnormality in four of our patients suggested the presence of a subtle underlying defect in energy metabolism.

Patients with alternating hemiplegia often have associated movement disorders consisting of choreoathetosis or dystonia. Some of the symptoms, particularly persistent hypotonia and paroxysmal dystonia may be prominent initially and later become less striking. Permanent dystonia, chorea, or choreoathetosis then supervene. Familial paroxysmal kinesigenic choreoathetosis may be considered in the differential diagnosis. It is however a distinct clinical syndrome not likely to be confused with alternating hemiplegia of childhood. It is not associated with hemiplegic attacks nor with psychomotor deterioration (18).

The recent international classification of headache (1988) has appropriately included alternating hemiplegia as a childhood periodic syndrome which might be associated with migraine (19). The relationship of alternating hemiplegia to migraine is strong (1,2,4). In our study 9 of the 10 patients had at least one first degree relative with a history of migraine. The early manifestations of the hemiplegic attacks are often accompanied by painful screaming, and by autonomic changes. Our patients frequently had attacks provoked by exposure to bright lights, by increased activity, or by excitement, and the episodes were frequently and perhaps always terminated by sleep. These clinical features are commonly associated with migraine. Patient 7 who has had gradual improvement in her language development over the years, can describe her attacks as starting with an aura of prickling sensation going up her arm and leg lasting for about 10 minutes followed by the hemiplegia. She had this aura bilaterally at the beginning of her generalized attacks. Afterward she had a severe throbbing headache, lasting most of the day, accompanied by nausea, pallor, photophobia, and sonophobia. She wanted to lie in a quiet, dark room and recovered after a brief sleep. The history of this more alert and observant patient suggested the possibility of a migrainous march. (J. Stephenson, *personal communication*, 1991) and Hockaday (3) have reported unusual patients with a similar history.

The evidence for a specific etiology of alternating hemiplegia of childhood is not conclusive. Studies of vascular function are ambiguous but they correlate with the absence of lesions attributable to stroke and with the fact that permanent hemiplegia does not develop over time. Cerebral vascular hypoperfusion might not adequately explain the clinical findings in alternating hemiplegia. The presence of a positive family history of migraine in parents needs to be confirmed in other series; the variability in the diagnosis of migraine by different physicians and even by neurologists is notorious. The symptomatology however is *sui generis*, and not identical to that of patients with sporadic or dominantly inherited hemiplegic migraine. The pain and misery of the children at the onset and the hint of a migrainous march in brighter affected individuals are however quite suggestive. Recent studies point to a trigeminovascular disturbance as the underlying basis for migraine (20). In addition there is an increase of glutamate in the cerebral cortex. These changes might be responsible for the spreading depression of Leao, for migraine, and perhaps also for alternating hemiplegia (21). The emergence of a persistent movement disorder suggests permanent damage to the basal ganglia. At present the main clue to the etiology is the abnormality found by MRS (see Chapter 20) but the cause and mechanism of the disorder still eludes us.

REFERENCES

1. Verret S, Steele JC. Alternating hemiplegia in childhood; A report of eight patients with complicated migraine beginning in infancy. *Pediatrics* 1971;47:675–680.
2. Hosking GP, Cavanagh NPC, Wilson J. Alternating hemiplegia: Complicated migraine of infancy. *Arch Dis Child* 1978;53:656–659.
3. Hockaday JM. Basilar artery migraine in childhood. *Dev Med Child Neurol* 1979;21:455–463.
4. Golden GH, French JH. Basilar artery migraine in young children. *Pediatrics* 1975;56:722–726.
5. Dittrich J, Havlóva M, Nevšímalová S. Paroxysmal hemiparesis of childhood. *Dev Med Child Neurol* 1979;21:800–807.
6. Krägeloh I, Aicardi J. Alternating hemiplegia in infants: Report of five cases. *Dev Med Child Neurol* 1980;22:784–791.
7. Dalla Bernardina B, Capovilla G, Trevisan E, et al. Alternating hemiplegia of childhood. In: Andermann F, Lugaresi E, eds. Migraine and epilepsy. London: Butterworths; 1987.
8. Aicardi J. Alternating hemiplegia of childhood. *Int Pediatr* 1987;2:115–119.

9. Andermann F, Silver K, St. Hilaire MH. Paroxysmal alternating hemiplegia of childhood: Treatment with flunarizine and other agents. *Neurology* 1986;36:327 (abst).
10. Myles ST, Needham CW, Leblanc FE. Alternating hemiparesis associated with hereditary hemorrhagic telangiectasia. *Can Med Assoc J* 1970;103:509–511.
11. Mikati M, Maguire H, Barlow FC, Bassett N, Treves TS. A new autosomal dominant syndrome of alternating hemiplegia of childhood: Chromosomal and physiological studies. *Ann Neurol* 1990; 28:416 (abst).
12. Kanazawa O, Shirasaka Y, Hattori H, Okuno T, Mikawa H. Ictal ^{99m}Tc-HMPAO SPECT in alternating hemiplegia. *Pediatr Neurol* 1991;7:2:121–124.
13. Zupanc ML, Dobkin JA, Perlman SB. ^{123}I-iodoamphetamine SPECT brain imaging in alternating hemiplegia. *Pediatr Neurol* 1991;7:1:35–38.
14. Paltiel HJ, O'Gorman M, Meagher-Villemure K, Rosenblatt B, Silver K, Watters GV. Subacute necrotizing encephalomyelopathy (Leigh's disease): CT Study. *Radiology* 1987;162:115–118.
15. Matthews PM, Tampieri D, Andermann F, Silver K, Arnold DL, Chitayat D. Magnetic resonance imaging shows specific abnormalities in the Melas syndrome. *Neurology* 1991;41:1043.
16. Lamoureux D, Silver K, Hodgkinson K, Chitayat D, Goodyer P. Spectrum of mitochondrial encephalomyopathies. *Can J Neurol Sci* 1991;18:22 (abst).
17. DiMauro S, Bonilla E, Lombes A, Shanske S, Minetti C, Moraes CT. Mitochondrial encephalomyopathies. In: Bodensteiner J, ed. Neurologic clinics. Philadelphia: WB Saunders; 1990;8: 3:483–506.
18. Lance JW. Familial paroxysmal dystonic choreoathetosis and its differentiation from related syndromes. *Ann Neurol* 1977;2:285–293.
19. Olesen J. Classification and diagnostic criteria for headache disorders. *Cephalalgia* 1988;8:[Suppl 7].
20. Moskowitz M. Basic mechanism in vascular headache. In: Mathew N, ed. Neurologic clinics. Philadelphia: WB Saunders; 1990;8:4:801–815.
21. Welch KMA, D'Anrea G, Tepley N, Barkley G, Ramadan M. Basic mechanism in vascular headache. In: Mathew N, ed. Neurologic clinics. Philadelphia: WB Saunders; 1990;8:4:817–828.

Alternating Hemiplegia of Childhood, edited by
Frederick Andermann, Jean Aicardi, and Federico Vigevano,
Raven Press, Ltd., New York © 1995.

3

Alternating Hemiplegia of Childhood: Clinical Findings During Attacks

Lucia Fusco and Federico Vigevano

*Section of Neurophysiology, "Bambino Gesù" Children's Hospital,
Piazza S. Onofrio, 4, 00165 Rome, Italy.*

This chapter focuses on the clinical description of the paroxysmal attacks in the alternating hemiplegia syndrome. Our observations are based on the ictal video/EEG recordings of six children with this disorder, recorded between the ages of 4 months and 5 years. Four children have been followed in our department since the onset of the disease and have undergone several ictal and interictal video/EEG recordings. In the other two children, recordings were obtained during a hemiplegic attack that occurred by chance during a consultation.

The patients described in the literature had heterogeneous clinical pictures. Several papers, which focused mainly on therapy or on investigation, referred generically to "typical" clinical symptoms, without further specification (1–4). Others described the clinical picture simply as hemiplegia (5–7). Fifty-four patients, described in greater detail (Table 1), had attacks that were referred to as unilateral, bilateral, or with features of both; the hemiplegia shifting from one side to the other (8–17). The alternating form is most frequently reported. At the onset or during the attack, 17 patients had eye movement abnormalities with eye deviation and horizontal nystagmus, as well as paralysis. Eight patients had monocular nystagmus. Some patients had tonic attacks during or outside the hemiplegic episodes. These generally started during the first year of life before the onset of the other symptoms.

MATERIAL AND METHODS

Four children (patients 1–4 in Table 2) were observed at our department from the beginning of the disease; in the other two, attacks were recorded during a consultation.

The six children ranged in age between 3 years 6 months and 7 years 8 months (mean 5 years 7 months). The age at onset of hemiplegic attacks ranged from 3

TABLE 1. *AHC: Patients described in detail*

Verret and Steele (1971)	3 (Patients 1,2,and 3)
Golden and French (1975)	1 (Patient 3)
Hosking et al. (1978)	6
Hockaday (1979)	1 (Patient 2)
Dittrich et al. (1979)	3
Aicardi (1980; with Krägeloh, 1987)	11
Dalla Bernardina et al. (1987)	3
Zupanc et al. (1991)	1
Mikati et al. (1992)	5
Silver and Andermann (1993)	10

months to 22 months (mean 9 months). The follow-up of the first four children was between 2 and 6 years (mean 3 years and 7 months) (Table 2).

Attacks recurred in all children with variable frequency, ranging from one a month to one a day. They lasted from several hours to 3 days, and in all children remitted as a consequence of sleep.

Two patients also had partial epileptic seizures. These attacks recurred rarely and were well controlled with antiepileptic drugs. All patients had delayed neurological development. Dystonic and dyskinetic features appeared during the second year of life. All the children had normal neuroimaging findings (MR and CT scan in all, and PET scan in two).

All children underwent video/EEG recording during the ictal and interictal phase. In the four children followed by us, several ictal recordings were obtained during different attacks.

RESULTS

Based on these recordings we were able to distinguish three types of hemiplegic attacks: unilateral, shifting, and bilateral. Some children had all three. In unilateral attacks the paralysis began and ended on the same side. In shifting attacks it began on one side, then shifted to the other, or finished on one side and continued on the other. In bilateral attacks both sides were usually paralyzed concurrently and equally. Shifting attacks and bilateral attacks appeared to be very similar events. Many bilateral attacks remained symmetrical only briefly. More often, the paralysis appeared to shift during the attack from one side to the other.

In these recordings, patients 1 and 5 had unilateral attacks; patients 1, 2, 3, and 6 had bilateral attacks; and patients 1 and 4 had shifting attacks. Recordings of patient 1 included unilateral, bilateral, and shifting attacks. Patient 2 had more than one ictal recording, all during bilateral attacks, the only type he had. Patient 3 also had several ictal video/EEG recordings; all showed bilateral paralysis. Patient 4 had several video/EEG recordings, but only one of them captured an attack consisting of ictal shifting paralysis. Patients 5 and 6 underwent recording once; patient 5 had a unilateral attack, and patient 6 a bilateral one.

TABLE 2. Clinical features of six patients with AHC

Patient no./Sex	Present age	Age at onset (OP)	Age at onset (AHC)	Type of paralysis Unilateral (a)	Bilateral (b)	Mixed (c)	Recorded attacks	Gaze dysfunction	Head/eye deviation	Tonic attacks
1/F	4 yr	45 days	7 mo	Yes	Yes	Yes	a,b,c	Yes	Yes	Yes
2/M	3 yr 6 mo	3 mo	6 mo	No	Yes	No	b	No	No	Yes
3/F	6 yr 6 mo	40 days	22 mo	No	Yes	No	b	Yes	No	Yes
4/M	6 yr 6 mo		7 mo	No	Yes	Yes	b,c	No	No	No
5/M	7 yr 8 mo	40 days	9 mo	Yes	?	?	a	Yes	Yes	Yes
6/M	6 yr 3 mo	3 mo	3 mo	Yes	Yes	No	b	Yes	No	No

OP, other paroxysmal phenomena (see text).

Clinical Features

The three types of hemiplegic attacks usually began with similar clinical symptoms, particularly yawning and drowsiness. The children looked exhausted and tired. These symptoms preceded the onset of the hemiplegia by 10 minutes or more.

Most hemiplegic attacks were accompanied by increased salivation, and by irregular and noisy breathing. These signs were particularly noticeable during bilateral paralysis.

Unilateral Attacks

During a unilateral attack, lack of movement was noted on one side, and ultimately ended in paralysis, which persisted until the end of the attack. The other side remained uninvolved and the child was able to move those limbs well (Fig. 1A). Unilateral attacks did not affect the facial muscles and the child was able to smile, cry, and talk (Fig. 1B).

Muscle tone varied: hypertonia and hypotonia could be observed in the same child during the same attack. Paralysis fluctuated over time and changed in intensity within a few seconds. At times the children seemed fatigued and motor performance worsened, but after a few minutes' rest, they were again able to move the affected limbs. When the movement returned, motor control was at first uncertain and movements hesitating and unsustained. Paralysis lasted hours and remitted with sleep. Pyramidal signs such as hyperreflexia or the Babinski sign were not present during the hemiplegia.

During a unilateral attack, hemiplegia was sometimes accompanied by other paroxysmal manifestations which were short, lasting from 2 to 6 minutes. They recurred several times during a single episode and consisted of four distinct phenomena:

1. Unilateral deviation of the eyes to the hemiparetic side (Fig. 1C); deviation was sometimes isolated, sometimes associated with head deviation. These two signs never followed a constant sequence (first eye then head deviation, or the reverse); they always happened at random.
2. Head deviation to the hemiplegic side, which was often associated with hyperextension of the neck (Fig. 1D). Previous reports have always referred to this sign as "head deviation." Close observation showed that this was not the tonic deviation observed in epileptic seizures but more a sideways movement of the head, or a tilting to one side like that observed in dystonic attacks or in torticollis. This head posture was not usually fixed; if strongly stimulated, the child could move the head back to its original position.
3. Complex lateral gaze dysfunction that most reports have described as monocular nystagmus. Although the more striking feature was nystagmus of one eye, close observation also disclosed impairment of movement of the contralateral eyeball. It remained fixed on the horizontal axis and would not move at all laterally but

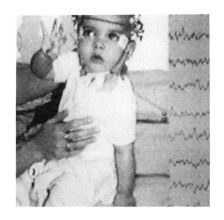

A

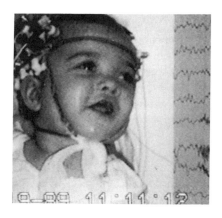

B

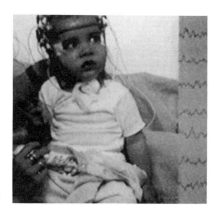

C

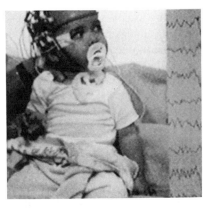

D

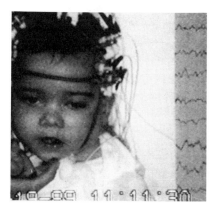

E

FIG. 1. This photo sequence shows patient 1, during a unilateral attack limited to the left side, at the age of 7 months and 15 days. **A:** The child is able to move the right arm, spontaneously or in response to stimulation. **B:** The face does not seem to be involved, and the child is able to smile symmetrically. **C:** Deviation of the eyes to the hemiparetic side occurs as an intermittent paroxysmal phenomenon. **D:** The lateral deviation of the eyes is at times associated with head deviation or tilting to the hemiparetic side. **E:** Detail during monocular nystagmus. The left eye is externally deviated, intermittently, at a rate of 1.5 to 2 beats per second. The right eye is fixed in the horizontal plane but vertical movements are possible.

could move vertically. The eye which showed nystagmus was partially or completely abducted with a lateral, arrhythmic, variable amplitude jerking (Fig. 1E). The child could not make other eye movements and the nystagmus was always unilateral. This type of gaze dysfunction was transient, and lasted from 1 to 10 minutes; the ocular symptoms ended spontaneously, and the eye movements then returned to normal.

Bilateral Attacks

A bilateral attack typically began with neck hypotonia, followed by upper trunk muscle weakness, limb hypotonia, and lack of movement (Fig. 2A–C). This sequence lasted several minutes and, for 10 minutes or more, the neck hypotonia could remain the only sign. However, once the process began it invariably led to complete paralysis. The attack was heralded by frequent yawns and plaintive behavior, and was commonly accompanied by hypersalivation, as well as irregular and noisy breathing. In patient 2, irregular breathing warned the parents that an attack was about to begin. Most children had difficulty swallowing and eating. Despite severe facial amimia, involuntary facial movements were usually unaffected

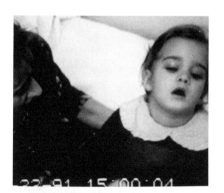

A

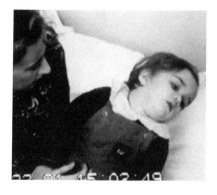

B

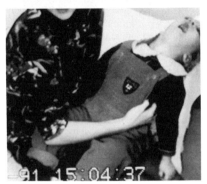

C

FIG. 2. The same child as in Fig. 1, at the onset of a bilateral attack. Paralysis begins with neck muscle hypotonia **(A)**, proceeds to upper trunk weakness **(B)**, and reduced limb movement **(C)**.

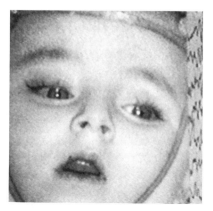
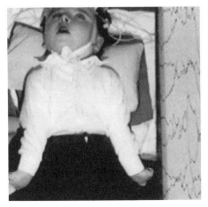

A   B

FIG. 3. Patient 2, during a bilateral attack. Note the absence of facial expression **(A)**, and the tonic attack in response to stimulation **(B)**.

(Fig. 3A). Spontaneous blinking was reduced and the blink reflex was inextinguishable. Ocular motility remained almost normal, although lateral eye movements were abnormally slow. In patients 3 and 4 convergent strabismus, present before their attacks, worsened. We never observed unilateral eye and head deviation, or lateral conjugate gaze dysfunction in a bilateral attack, even when the attack began with unilaterally diminished movements. At times other paroxysmal phenomena, such as tonic stiffening and a dystonic posture occurred spontaneously or could be provoked by stimulating the patient (see below). Pyramidal signs such as the Babinski sign, hyperreflexia, or hypertonia were difficult to evaluate: two patients who manifested these signs during attacks also had them in the interictal period.

The paralysis disappeared during sleep, so that on waking, the child was generally symptom free. During a bilateral attack, the paralysis sometimes fluctuated in severity, affecting one side predominantly, or varying in maximal severity from one side to the other.

Shifting Attacks

We defined "shifting" attacks as those in which paralysis began on one side and shifted to the other, without recovery in between. The lack of movement shifted from one side to the other, and the recovery began on one side. During most of a shifting attack the paralysis was almost completely confined to one side. Yet in shifting attacks we never observed the focal paroxysmal phenomena that accompanied unilateral attacks. On the contrary, most of their features suggested that a shifting attack was an abortive bilateral attack in which the weakness from time to time predominated on one side. The manifestations typically observed in shifting attacks—loss of facial expression, difficulty in swallowing and eating—were those seen in bilateral attacks.

Tonic Attacks

Although many parents clearly described focal or diffuse tonic episodes occurring during or outside the attacks of paralysis, we recorded tonic attacks only in patient 2. In this child, tonic stiffening occurred in response to vigorous stimulation during bilateral attacks (Fig. 3B). These tonic episodes were characterized by paroxysmal hyperextension of the limbs lasting several seconds. They occurred in series that continued for several minutes, always in response to the stimulus.

EEG Features

Even though focal abnormalities were never present during unilateral or bilateral attacks, neither were the EEGs completely normal. Especially during bilateral episodes, the recordings showed a pattern of 6 to 7 Hz theta activity, which was either diffuse or predominated over the central vertex (Fig. 4A). Stimuli evoking tonic fits caused desynchronization of the theta pattern (Fig. 4B), which probably represented an arousal reaction. None of the children ever had EEG abnormalities during sleep (Fig. 5), not even during sleep that followed a hemiplegic attack. In patient 4 the attack stopped after a brief rest, which corresponded on the EEG to transient drowsiness, without the synchronization and the physiological discharges characteristic of sleep.

DISCUSSION

In attempting to localize the brain dysfunction responsible for the hemiplegic phenomenon described in these children, a detailed analysis of the symptoms can be of great help. The first step consists of analyzing the weakness itself. In our patients, apart from the paralysis, associated more often with hypotonia than with hypertonia, signs pointing to a strictly pyramidal localization—hyperreflexia, the Babinski sign, a facilitation or spread of the area giving rise to the reflex were notably absent. Muscle tone provided no diagnostic help: our patients had both hypotonia and hypertonia.

In contrast to the absence of pyramidal signs, the patients showed clear evidence for extrapyramidal and cerebellar dysfunction—more obvious and noticeable in patients with incomplete paralysis. They had difficulty initiating movements, a form of motor inertia or bradykinesia. Once initiated, the movements were executed slowly, inaccurately, and often with an unsteadiness recalling dysmetria. The apparent sparing of the facial musculature in unilateral attacks provides further evidence of extrapyramidal or cerebellar dysfunction. Another distinctive feature was fatigability, that improved after rest.

The gaze dysfunction recorded during unilateral attacks is reminiscent of the "one-and-a-half" syndrome, an unusual internuclear ophthalmoplegia that combines two deficits of horizontal eye movements. Lateral conjugate palsy in one direction

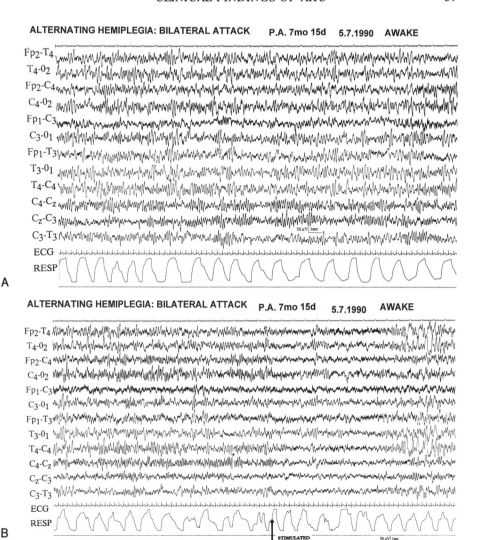

FIG. 4. A: EEG recording of patient 2 during the attack illustrated in Fig. 3A; diffuse theta activity at 6 Hz is evident, better organized over the vertex. **B:** After vigorous voice stimulation, a tonic attack is recorded (Fig. 3B) corresponding to desynchronization of the EEG.

(one) and adduction paralysis in the other direction (and-a-half) are present. In the complete form of the syndrome one eye cannot deviate laterally from the midline and the other eye can only be abducted from the midline. Unilateral nystagmus of the abducted eye becomes evident when the eyes attempt to deviate to the side contralateral to the gaze paralysis. Most vertical eye movements are preserved. If correct, the analogy with the neuro-ophthalmologic signs of the one-and-a-half syn-

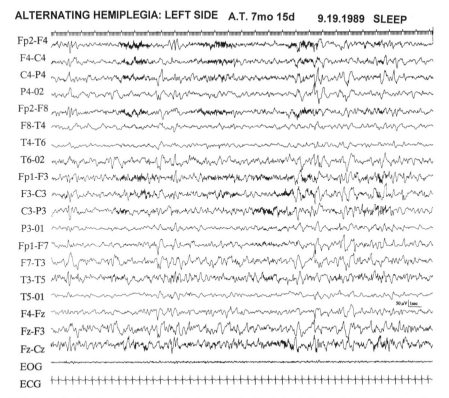

FIG. 5. Patient 1. Sleep EEG recording during a left-sided attack. Phase II: Diffuse theta pattern, K-complexes and spindles are well formed.

drome implies damage to the dorsal tegmentum in the lower pons, the area held responsible for the complete syndrome (18,19). Yet it does not explain why the many known variants of the syndrome are lesional in origin (19), whereas the symptoms accompanying attacks of unilateral paralysis seem to reflect a transient dysfunction. Whatever the explanation, the one-and-a-half syndrome is the only neurological disorder manifesting with unilateral nystagmus of known anatomic location. The damaged brain structures in the one-and-a-half syndrome are the parapontine nucleus, which controls lateral conjugate gaze, and the medial longitudinal fasciculus, which controls adduction of the ipsilateral eye.

Tonic eye deviation, a common sign during unilateral attacks, could be of cortical origin, but could also result from an abnormality of parapontine lateral conjugate gaze control, where a lesion is known to provoke ipsilateral conjugate deviation (20).

The head deviation in our patients recalls that observed in paroxysmal torticollis and particularly resembles that of spasmus nutans. Spasmus nutans is a benign, usually self-limiting condition, with onset in the first year of life and disappearance within the second year (21). It often remains undiagnosed. The three characteristic signs are head nodding, head tilt, and nystagmus. Atypical cases have been described that are symptomatic of a hypothalamic and diencephalic lesion (22). Patients with typical spasmus nutans commonly have monocular nystagmus (21). Nystagmus, most frequently the unilateral form, and head tilt are the two characteristic signs of this syndrome. Even though its localization and pathogenesis remain unclear, much evidence points to a dysfunction of the vestibular nuclei in the brainstem (21).

The signs that precede or accompany attacks of alternating hemiplegia—yawning, hypersalivation, and difficulty swallowing—also suggest brainstem involvement.

Finally, the EEG pattern, characterized by nonspecific monomorphic theta wave activity, reflects the rhythms characteristic of brainstem or pontine dysfunction.

In conclusion, our analysis of the clinical features observed during attacks of alternating hemiplegia in these children suggests involvement of the mesencephalic and pontine structures. This localization is further confirmed by the lack of EEG signs attributable to hemispheric compromise and by the presence of rhythms compatible with brainstem involvement.

Analyzing how the attacks changed over time proved to be of interest. Patient 1 was the only one who had all three types of attacks and at a certain stage in her life these coexisted. Figure 6 clearly shows that the paroxysmal motor phenomena of head and/or eye deviation and of conjugate gaze dysfunction nearly always occurred during unilateral attacks, and that both phenomena diminished during the first year of life. As unilateral attacks diminished in frequency, bilateral or shifting attacks became more frequent. These last two types generally had no associated paroxysmal motor phenomena. Unilateral attacks and paroxysmal phenomena may simply reflect the younger age and less mature brain at the time when they occur.

Persistently unilateral attacks occurred more rarely; we only observed them in two of the six children in our series. It is difficult to say whether they correlated with less severe disease. In patient 1, the onset of bilateral attacks corresponded with clinical worsening of the pre-existing dystonic syndrome. The four patients who had only bilateral or shifting attacks from the onset were clinically no worse than those who had had strictly unilateral attacks. The severity of the disease did not correlate with the type of attack present at the onset of symptoms nor with early onset (Table 2).

Patient 4, whose attacks started at 7 months of age, was almost normal neurologically between attacks, whereas patient 3, whose attacks started at the age of 22 months, had marked dystonic symptoms, even though she managed to walk unaided. This confirms the importance of the other features of the neurological syndrome. The presence of associated epilepsy, for example, as in patient 3, might be responsible for more severe clinical manifestations, independent of the age of onset of the attacks.

The attacks of paralysis have always been the major clinical feature because the disability associated with them has such an impact on the patient's daily life. For this reason they have led to recognition of the syndrome and have been identified with it. Our impression is that they are mere epiphenomena of a more complex

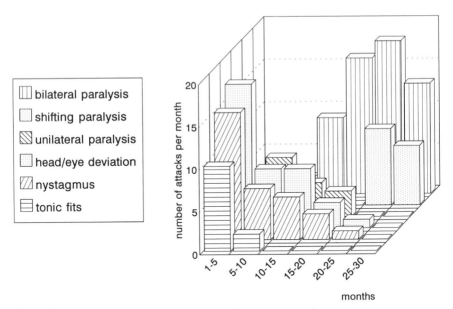

FIG. 6. Occurrence of the different paroxysmal phenomena over time.

neurological disease encompassing multisystem dysfunction. The anatomical and biochemical correlates of this disease, however, have yet to be identified.

REFERENCES

1. Casaer P, Azou M. Flunarizine in alternating hemiplegia in childhood. [Letter]. *Lancet* 1984;2:579.
2. Salmon MA, Wilson J. Drugs for alternating hemiplegic migraine. [Letter]. *Lancet* 1984;2:980.
3. Siemes H. Rectal chloral hydrate for alternating hemiplegia of childhood. [Letter]. *Dev Med Child Neurol* 1990;32:927–931.
4. Andermann F, Silver K, St.-Hilaire MH, et al. Paroxysmal alternating hemiplegia of childhood: treatment with flunarizine and other agents. *Neurology* 1986;36:327 (abst).
5. Santanelli P, Guerrini R, Dravet C, Genton P, Bureau M, Farnarier G. Brainstem auditory evoked potentials in alternating hemiplegia: ictal vs. interictal assessment in one case. *Clinical EEG* 1990; 21:51–54.
6. Kanazawa O, Shirasaka Y, Hattori H, Okuno T, Mikawa H. Ictal ^{99m}Tc-HMPAO SPECT in alternating hemiplegia. *Pediatr Neurol* 1991;7:121–124.
7. Siemes H, Casaer P. Alternating hemiplegia in childhood: a clinical report and single photon emission computed tomography study. *Monatsschr Kinderheilkd* 1988;136:467–470.
8. Verret S, Steele JC. Alternating hemiplegia in childhood: a report of eight patients with complicated migraine beginning in infancy. *Pediatrics* 1971;47:675–680.
9. Golden GS, French JH. Basilar migraine in young children. *Pediatrics* 1975;56:722–726.
10. Hosking GP, Cavanagh NPC, Wilson J. Alternating hemiplegia: complicated migraine of infancy. *Arch Dis Child* 1978;53:656–659.
11. Dittrich J, Havlová M, Nevsímalová S. Paroxysmal hemiparesis in childhood. *Dev Med Child Neurol* 1979;21:800–807.
12. Aicardi J. Alternating hemiplegia of childhood. *Int Pediatr* 1987;2:115–119.
13. Krägeloh I, Aicardi J. Alternating hemiplegia in infants: report of five cases. *Dev Med Child Neurol* 1980;22:784–791.

14. Dalla Bernardina B, Capovilla G, Trevisan E, et al. Alternating hemiplegia in childhood. In: Andermann F, Lugaresi E, eds. *Migraine and epilepsy.* Butterworths; 1987;189–201.
15. Zupanc ML, Dobkin JA, Perlman SB. ^{123}I-iodoamphetamine SPECT brain imaging in alternating hemiplegia. *Pediatr Neurol* 1991;7:35–38.
16. Mikati MA, Maguire H, Barlow CF, et al. A syndrome of autosomal dominant alternating hemiplegia: clinical presentation mimicking intractable epilepsy; chromosomal study; and physiologic investigations. *Neurology* 1992;42:2251–2257.
17. Silver K, Andermann F. Alternating hemiplegia of childhood: a study of 10 patients and results of flunarizine treatment. *Neurology* 1993;43:36–41.
18. Fisher CM. Some neuro-ophthalomological observations. *J Neurol Neurosurg Psychiatry* 1967; 30:383–392.
19. Pierrot-Deseilligny Ch, Chain F, Serdaru M, Gray F, Lhermitte F. The 'one-and-a-half' syndrome. Electro-oculographic analysis of five cases with deductions about the physiological mechanism of lateral gaze. *Brain* 1981;104:665–699.
20. Cohen B, Komatsuzaki A. Eye movements induced by stimulation of the pontine reticular formation: evidence for integration in oculomotor pathways. *Exp Neurol* 1972;36:101–117.
21. Jayalakshmi P, McNair Scott TF, Tucker SH, Schaffer DB. Infantile nystagmus: a prospective study of spasmus nutans, congenital nystagmus, and unclassified nystagmus of infancy. *J Pediatr* 1970; 77:177–187.
22. Antony JH, Ouvrier RA, Wise G. Spasmus nutans: A mistaken identity. *Arch Neurol* 1980;37:373–375.

Alternating Hemiplegia of Childhood, edited by
Frederick Andermann, Jean Aicardi, and Federico Vigevano,
Raven Press, Ltd., New York © 1995.

4

Clinical Findings in 23 Japanese Patients with Alternating Hemiplegia of Childhood

Norio Sakuragawa

Department of Inherited Metabolic Diseases, National Institute of Neuroscience, National Center for Neurology and Psychiatry, 4-1-1, Ogawahigashi-cho, Kodaira, Tokyo, 187 Japan.

Alternating hemiplegia of childhood (AHC) is a rare disorder with characteristic clinical features. In 1988, a large Japanese cooperative study was carried out which identified 23 patients with AHC (1,2). In all, at least 58 patients have been described in the literature up to 1988. This disorder may be more common or more often recognized and reported in Japan than in western countries. This report is aimed to clarify whether any differences in clinical features exist between Japanese patients and those from other countries.

COMPARISON OF CLINICAL FEATURES DESCRIBED IN JAPAN AND IN WESTERN COUNTRIES

The clinical characteristics of this disorder in Japanese patients are shown in Table 1. Table 2 presents a comparison between AHC in Japan and reported patients (3,8) from western countries regarding histories, clinical symptoms, and laboratory data. A family history of migraine was infrequently obtained in Japan. Perinatal abnormal histories were higher in Japan: 61% of patients had a history of abnormality such as neonatal asphyxia due to respiratory distress syndrome, cesarean section due to placenta praevia, cephalo-pelvic disproportion, neonatal jaundice, etc. Developmental milestones were usually delayed in Japanese children (78% of patients in Japan and 42% in western countries). However, a recent report from Canada (8) indicated that 7 out of 8 patients were globally delayed.

The typical presentation of attacks does not differ in Japan and western countries (1,8), indicating that the clinical entity is similar. The core sign is the repetitive occurrence of episodes of flaccid hemiplegia or bilateral hemiplegic attacks, manifested by generalized flaccidity. There are also several additional characteristic signs which delineate this clinical entity. Prodromes of attacks observed in 68% of

43

TABLE 1. *Clinical characteristics of AHC in Japan*

1. No difference according to sex.
2. Unremarkable findings in family history.
3. The peak of onset of hemiplegic episodes was between 5 and 9 months of age.
4. Hemiplegia was usually flaccid in nature but sometimes spastic, and at times affected both sides of the body.
5. Prodromes or precipitating factors for hemiplegia were present and characteristic. Rest and sleep were effective for recovery.
6. Hemiplegic episodes were frequently associated with other neurological abnormalities.
7. Mental and neurological abnormalities became manifest in the early stages of this disorder or were present even prior to the onset of hemiplegic attacks.
8. Developmental progress was seen, although the children were usually retarded.
9. Atypical cases may be present: normal early psychomotor development or onset later than 18 months of age.

TABLE 2. *Comparison between AHC in Japan and reported cases in western countries: histories, clinical symptoms, and main laboratory data*

	Japanese AHC (n = 23)	Western AHC (n = 35)
Sex, male:female	12:11	20:11
	(23)	(54)
Migraine in family history	9.1%	47%
	(2/22)	(9/19)
Abnormal pregnancy histories	8.7%	5.3%
	(2/23)	(1/19)
Abnormal perinatal histories	61%	11%
	(14/23)	(2/19)
Delayed milestones	78%	42%
	(18/23)	(8/19)
Neurological abnormalities[a]		
Mental retardation	87%	100%
	(20/23)	(17/17)
Involuntary movements	48%	44%
	(11/23)	(11/25)
Hypotonia	57%	21%
	(13/23)	(4/19)
Ataxia	22%	11%
	(5/23)	(2/19)
Convulsions	59%	47%
	(13/22)	(9/19)
Abnormal EEG[b]	45%	68%
	(10/22)	(13/19)
Abnormal CT	13%	0%
	(3/23)	(0/6)

[a]Neurological abnormality between hemiplegic attacks.
[b]Abnormal EEG during and between hemiplegic attacks.
n, total number of cases.

Japanese patients included temper tantrums, headaches, hyperpnea, and autonomic nervous symptoms (Fig. 1). Seventy-eight percent of patients in western countries had similar prodromes such as screaming, restlessness, etc. Provoking factors were reported in 60% of Japanese patients (Fig. 2). Similarly, 70% to 75% of the patients reported by Silver and Andermann (3) had attacks triggered by exposure to bright light, excitement, bathing, loud noises, specific food, or anti-convulsant medication.

Neurological examination between hemiplegic attacks showed abnormalities similar to those reported from the West: hypotonia, ataxia, and involuntary movements. Half to 60% of patients developed epileptic seizures in Japan, Europe, and North America, usually generalized and well controlled by medication.

LABORATORY STUDIES

Extensive laboratory investigations did not reveal any diagnostic abnormality. Studies included CT, MRI, PET, SPECT, ABR and SER, and muscle or liver biopsies searching for evidence of mitochondrial disturbance. Contralateral EEG slowing without epileptiform discharges was observed during attacks in about half the patients. Chromosome analysis was normal in three patients reported by Silver and Andermann (8). Mikati et al. (9,10) recently reported an autosomal dominant syndrome of AHC. Their patients showed a chromosomal abnormality: t(3;9) (p26;q34). One Japanese patient, who had the clinical criteria of AHC, had a chromosomal abnormality identified as 46 XX,t(7;16)(q11;23) (Takakusaki, *personal communication*, 1990).

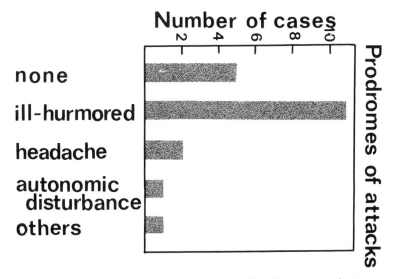

FIG. 1. Prodromes of attacks were observed in 68% of Japanese patients.

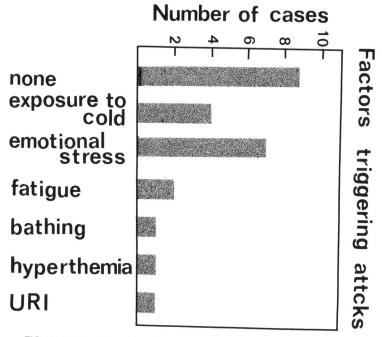

FIG. 2. Factors triggering attacks were reported in 60% of Japanese patients.

DISCUSSION

The etiological relationship between migraine and AHC has been pointed out early. A family history of migraine is prominent in western countries. Silver and Andermann reported that 9 of their 10 patients had at least one first degree relative with a history of migraine (8). Such a history was not as frequent in Japan. However, Japanese patients (70%) frequently experienced a prodrome of temper tantrums, headaches, hyperpnea, and autonomic nervous symptoms. Patients in western countries had almost the same clinical features during the prodrome, manifestations which are commonly associated with migraine. These data strongly indicate that AHC might be associated with migraine.

The inheritance of this disorder has not yet been proven. There were no reports of affected siblings or first or second degree family members with other neurological disorders, alternating hemiplegia, or epilepsy (1,8). Recently Mikati et al. (9,10) described the first familial occurrence of this disorder with a balanced reciprocal translocation at 46XY,t(3;9)(p26;q34). Although this family seems to have a syndrome different from the usual form of AHC because of the autosomal dominant inheritance, more sophisticated investigation of chromosomal structures may throw some light on the nature of the sporadic disorder.

REFERENCES

1. Sakuragawa N. Alternating hemiplegia in childhood: 23 cases in Japan. *Brain Dev* 1992;14:283–288.
2. Sakuragawa N, Arima M, Matsumoto S. Nationwide investigation of alternating hemiplegia of children in Japan. *Nippon Shonika Gakka Zasshi (Tokyo)* 1988;92:892–898.
3. Verret S, Steele JC. Alternating hemiplegia in childhood: a report of 8 patients with complicated migraine beginning in infancy. *Pediatrics* 1971;47:675–680.
4. Golden GS, French JH. Basilar artery migraine in young children. *Pediatrics* 1975;56:722–726.
5. Hosking GP, Cavanagh NPC, Wilson J. Alternating hemiplegia: complicated migraine of infancy. *Arch Dis Child* 1979;53:656–659.
6. Hockaday JM. Basilar artery migraine in childhood. *Dev Med Child Neurol* 1979;21:455–463.
7. Dittrich J, Havlóva M, Nevšímalová S. Paroxysmal hemiparesis in childhood. *Dev Med Child Neurol* 1979;21:800–807.
8. Silver K, Andermann F. Alternating hemiplegia of childhood: A study of 10 patients and results of flunarizine treatment. *Neurology* 1993.
9. Mikati M, Maguire H, Barlow CF, Bassett N, et al. A new autosomal dominant syndrome of alternating hemiplegia of childhood: Chromosomal and physiological studies. *Ann Neurol* 1990;28:416.
10. Mikati M, Ozelius L, Breakfield X, Klawck S, Korf B. Linkage analysis in autosomal-dominant alternating hemiplegia of childhood. *Ann Neurol* 1992;32:451.

Alternating Hemiplegia of Childhood, edited by
Frederick Andermann, Jean Aicardi, and Federico Vigevano,
Raven Press, Ltd., New York © 1995.

5

Alternating Hemiplegia of Childhood: Long-Term Outcome

Marie Bourgeois, *Soňa Nevšímalová, †Jean Aicardi, and
‡Frederick Andermann

*Department of Pediatrics, Hôpital des Enfants Malades, 149 rue de Sèvres, 75743 Paris
Cedex 15, France; *Department of Neurology, Charles University, Kateřinská 30, 120 00
Prague 2, Czech Republic; †Institute of Child Health, Mecklenburgh Square, University of
London, London WC1N 2AP, England; and ‡Departments of Neurology, Neurosurgery,
and Pediatrics, Montreal Neurological Hospital and Institute, 3801 University Street,
McGill University, Montreal, Quebec H3A 2B4, Canada.*

The short-term and middle-term course of alternating hemiplegia of childhood (AHC) has been well described. All the patients so far reported continue to present attacks of hemiplegia associated with tonic/dystonic attacks and often other paroxysmal phenomena such as nystagmus or strabismus (1–3). As the patients grow older, there may be a tendency for these associated features to become less prominent (4–6) although this has not been well documented. Virtually all children with the condition have neurodevelopmental difficulties and developmental delay. Mental retardation, and extrapyramidal features, especially choreoathetosis, are present after the age of 2 to 5 years (4,5).

The long-term outcome of AHC has not been specifically studied. We therefore report the cases of 10 patients followed up well into adolescence or early adulthood.

PATIENTS AND CLINICAL FINDINGS

There were three girls and seven boys ranging in age from 13 to 29 years at the time of last examination (Table 1). All had a typical history and demonstrated the characteristic features of the condition (see Chapter 1). Age at first attack varied between 3 days and 8 months and age at first hemiplegic episode was under 18 months in all cases. Five patients were seen at the Hôpital des Enfants Malades, Paris (see Chapter 1), four patients were followed up at the Neurological Clinic of Charles University, Prague, and one at the Montreal Neurological Hospital (see Chapter 2). All the patients underwent extensive diagnostic investigations including

TABLE 1. Long-term clinical findings

Patient no., sex, and age at end of follow-up (yrs)	Age at onset (months)		Initial development	Epileptic seizures (SZS)	Neurological findings[a]	Last mental assessment	Treatment with flunarizine from age, (yrs), duration (yrs), and result
	Of attacks	Of Episodes of hemiplegia					
1, M, 27	3	7	Slow, DQ-65 at 15 mo	?	ChA-At marked	Severe MR	—
2, F, 18	4	6	Normal	3 szs at 3, 7 and 9 yrs	ChA, marked dystonia	IQ = 60–70	7.5 / 1 / No effect
3, M, 14.8	3	3	Mildly delayed	2 szs at 14 yrs	ChA mild, At mild	IQ: untestable at 8s, autistic	6 / 8 / Partial effect
4, M,[a] 14.5	2	3	Normal	0	ChA, mild acquired hemiparesis	IQ<50	11 / 3.5 / No effect
5, M, 13	1	5	Normal but for hypotonia	0	ChA intense, At marked	IQ = 80	4 / 9 / Good effect
6, M, 29	8	14	Early hypotonia DQ = 75 at 2 yrs	Few szs between 7 and 8	ChA, mild hemiparesis	IQ = 40	28 / 1 / No effect
7, F, 26	4	8	Early hypotonia DQ = at 2 yrs	szs at 4 yrs	ChA, AT	IQ=38 at 16	25 / 1 / Some effect
8, M, 14 +	6	6	Markedly delayed	Sporadic szs	ChA, marked dystonia	IQ = 35	—
9, M, 16	0.4	12	Delayed	0	ChA, hemiparesis At	IQ<50	15 / 1 / Partial effect
10, F, 27	3	7	Normal	Severe from 7 yrs	ChA, At	IQ<40	19 / No effect

[a]Patient had two periods without paroxysmal episodes between ages 2 and 5 and 5.5 and 9 years.
At, ataxia; ChA, choreoathetosis; MR, mental retardation.

angiography and CT or MR scans in most, and no cause was found for their attacks. None of these patients had a family history of a similar disorder.

In most patients, initial development had seemed unremarkable for the first few months or the first year of life. However, one patient (patient 8) was obviously retarded from the outset and another one (patient 10) had had a "small head" from birth.

One patient (patient 8) died at age 14 years of bronchopneumonia that followed three "severe episodes of alternating hemiplegia." This child had profound mental retardation, marked hypotonia, extrapyramidal signs, stunted growth, and appeared to have had a very severe form of the disease.

The remaining nine patients continued to have frequent episodes of hemiplegia and, even in the oldest ones, there was no appreciable decrease in the frequency of attacks. Most of them also continued to suffer tonic or dystonic attacks that may have been uni- or bilateral and often intense and painful. In one of them (patient 3), the frequency of tonic attacks seemed to increase in recent years. In contrast, paroxysmal nystagmus disappeared in all cases before age 10 years.

Seven patients have had true epileptic attacks in addition to their hemiplegic and tonic attacks. Most seizures were generalized tonic-clonic or unilateral seizures. In one case, there was a suspicion of brief atypical absence seizures. The epilepsy was severe in some children (e.g., patient 10 had two severe episodes of status epilepticus requiring admission to an intensive care unit) while others had only occasional episodes, sometimes occurring at the peak of a hemiplegic attack (e.g., patient 3).

None of the patients developed typical migraine attacks. One patient complained of "pain in the eyes" before an attack; another one asked for aspirin but denied any headache.

Mental retardation was present at end of follow-up in all but two patients who had IQs of 80 (patients 3 and 5). One of these (patient 3) exhibited severe psychotic features. Another child (patient 2) was mildly retarded with an IQ of between 60 and 70. The remaining patients had IQs between 38 and 50 and most also exhibited behavioral problems. They were, however, relatively self-sufficient in everyday life but were dependent on family or institutional care.

All affected persons were ambulant at end of follow-up although their gait was usually ataxic and interfered with by choreic or choreoathetotic movements. Language was limited to simple sentences with a restricted vocabulary in most cases. However, the two patients with the highest IQ also had well developed language even though they were sometimes difficult to understand because of marked dysarthria. Only these two patients had relatively normal schooling but showed increasing difficulties at the end of primary school.

All affected patients had severe neurological abnormalities. The most common was choreoathetosis that usually appeared early in life, no later than at 5 years of age. In older patients, dystonia or hemidystonia was often superimposed. Cerebellar ataxia was also found in most patients and pyramidal tract signs, usually of a slight to moderate degree were common. Spasticity at times replaced the marked hypotonia that may be present at onset. Three children developed signs of persistent mild hemiparesis on the side most frequently involved by the paroxysmal attacks. This occurred as late as age 7 years in patient 4, who became left-handed after having had multiple right-sided episodes of hemiplegia. The degree of functional impairment was usually quite significant and walking was difficult due to ataxia and hypotonia. Choreoathetosis and/or dystonia prevented fine hand movements. Writing was not possible in the relatively high-functioning patients who had to use a typewriter.

All patients were small and underweight in early adulthood or late adolescence. Evidence of neurological and/or mental deterioration was clearly present in most cases (except in patient 8 who had severe developmental delay from the first days of life), as indicated by the contrast between findings at the last examination and normal or near normal performance during the first year of life. Neurological abnormalities such as hemiparesis, spasticity and especially choreoathetosis were clearly acquired, usually around 2 to 4 years of age. Mental deterioration, on the other hand, was more difficult to ascertain because of the young age at onset of the disorder, the often slow initial development, and because of the fluctuations that could have occurred in relation to the hemiplegic episodes. One of our patients (patient 8) had a measured IQ of 80 at 3 and 5 years of age, then of 60 at 7 years following a severe episode, and again of 80 at 8 years. There is little doubt, however, that in most patients there is an actual decline of IQ (e.g., from 75 to 40 in patient 6).

Episodes of obvious deterioration took place in most patients following severe bilateral paralytic and/or dystonic attacks. Previously acquired milestones such as walking and language could be lost for periods lasting from a few days to several months during which a severe IQ loss was also apparent. Recovery from such episodes seemed to be complete but could usually not be documented by repeated psychological testing.

Some evidence of actual progression of the disease could be inferred from the study of evoked potentials and of SPECT (single photon emission computed tomography) as the results of these examinations tended to be more abnormal in older patients than early in the course of the illness.

Three patients (patients 6, 7, and 9) had prolonged latency of the "cognitive evoked potential" P300; latency was 376 ms in patient 6 at 16 years of age and 480 ms in patient 7 aged 26 years. Similar changes were found in visual evoked potentials. The latency of P100 was normal only in the youngest patient (patient 9). In the 16-year-old patient, the response was atypical with increased temporal dispersion and mildly prolonged latency of P100, whilst in the 26-year-old girl, latency of P100 was clearly prolonged, up to 172 milliseconds. Brainstem auditory evoked responses on the other hand were normal in all patients tested.

SPECT demonstrated hypoperfusion of the affected hemisphere early in life during an attack of hemiplegia in patient 6, while in patient 7 mild signs of hypoperfusion were present in both parietal regions interictally during the third decade of life also suggesting increasingly abnormal brain function.

COMMENTS

The present study confirms earlier reports on the severity of AHC (1–6) and indicates that the disease remains active even after a prolonged course. In this series of patients, no significant decrease in the frequency and severity of the paroxysmal episodes was apparent after the illness had lasted 3 to almost 30 years. Indeed, the only change in the clinical symptomatology of attacks was the disappearance of abnormal eye movements before adolescence. Contrary to previous impression (5), tonic attacks and associated autonomic or respiratory features can persist into adolescence and early adulthood, at least in some patients. Likewise, involvement of pharyngeal-laryngeal muscles can persist during severe attacks and probably played an essential role in generating the pulmonary complications that led to the death of patient 8.

Cognitive deficit was present to some degree in all our patients and a progressive decline of IQ was observed in some children. It is difficult, however, to determine whether this was due to an actual loss of previously acquired skills or to an increasing discrepancy between developmental and chronological ages as a result of arrested progress. The overall clinical impression in most patients was that development was slow during the first two years of life, then became even slower over the next few years to finally reach a plateau before age 10. Such a course was particularly apparent in those individuals with highest mental function (patients 3 and 5) who seemed unable to make any further acquisitions after age 8 years. Nevertheless, actual regression with loss of skills cannot be excluded in the most severely affected children and progressive neurological deterioration is clearly present at least during the first three to five years of life manifested by the development of movement disorder and ataxia.

Study of evoked potentials and of SPECT also suggested progression of the disease as the more abnormal results were obtained in the oldest patients. However, longitudinal studies of very few patients are currently available and further studies are clearly indicated. Siemes and Cordes (6) recently reported that areas of hypoperfusion in one patient varied over time, without definite pattern.

The severity of the mental handicap is variable from profound retardation to low normal intelligence. Epilepsy is a common complicating feature and appears to become more frequent in older patients. It was present in seven of the patients described in this series and only in 6 of 22 patients of any age previously reported (5). No clear relationship is apparent between the severity of the neurological manifestations and that of the mental retardation as some of the highest functioning patients in this series had very severe choreoathetosis (e.g., patient 5). Severe epilepsy may have some relation to a poor mental outcome but occasional seizures do not seem to be important in this respect; however, the small number of patients limits the validity of this observation.

We have tried to determine whether early features of the condition could help predict the outcome but only tentative remarks can be offered.

The presence of early retardation, especially of marked hypotonia in the first months of life seemed to predict a severe course. Age at first attack was unrelated to outcome.

No clear relationship emerged between the frequency and severity of hemiplegic attacks and the degree of mental retardation. Thus, patient 5 had good mental function despite an extremely high frequency of attacks. Conversely, the occurrence of long periods of up to two years without attacks did not prevent severe retardation in patient 4. On the contrary, the occurrence of bilateral hemiplegias or of generalized dystonic attacks, especially when prolonged and severe was clearly correlated with a poor mental outcome. Such episodes were associated with profound regression with slow recovery. Despite apparently complete recovery following such episodes, the possibility exists that mild residua persisted after each attack, which might have been detected by detailed neuropsychological assessment. Accumulation of such minor residual deficits could in turn be one mechanism of progression of the disease in AHC.

Determining the effect of repeated attacks on outcome is of obvious practical importance as flunarizine, the only treatment currently available, is effective in lessening the severity and duration of the paroxysms, even though it usually does not greatly reduce their frequency (7,8). Unfortunately, the present study does not permit us to draw firm conclusions regarding the long-term effect of such treatment because most patients were treated late and not in a systematic manner. It seems reasonable, however, to believe that early and continued treatment could help lessen the devastating effect and improve the endpoint of this disease.

REFERENCES

1. Dittrich J, Havlóva M, Nevšímalová S. Paroxysmal hemiparesis of childhood. *Dev Med Child Neurol* 1979;21:800–807.
2. Krägeloh I, Aicardi J. Alternating hemiplegia in infants: report of five cases. *Dev Med Child Neurol* 1980;22:784–791.
3. Dalla Bernardina B, Capovilla G, Trevisan E et al. Alternating hemiplegia of infants. In: Andermann F, Lugaresi E, eds. *Migraine and epilepsy.* London: Butterworths; 1987:189–201.
4. Aicardi J. Alternating hemiplegia of childhood. *International Pediatrics* 1987;2:115–119.
5. Bourgeois M, Aicardi J, Goutières F. Alternating hemiplegia of childhood. *J Pediatr* 1993;122:673–679.
6. Siemes H, Cordes M. Single photon emission computed tomography investigations of alternating hemiplegia of childhood. *Dev Med Child Neurol* 1993;35:366–380.
7. Silver K, Andermann F. Alternating hemiplegia of childhood: a study of 10 patients and results of flunarizine treatment. *Neurology* 1993;43:36–41.
8. Casaer P. Flunarizine in alternating hemiplegia in childhood. An international study of 12 children. *Neuropediatrics* 1987;18:191–195.

Investigation of Patients with Alternating Hemiplegia of Childhood

Alternating Hemiplegia of Childhood, edited by
Frederick Andermann, Jean Aicardi, and Federico Vigevano,
Raven Press, Ltd., New York © 1995.

6

Alternating Hemiplegia of Childhood: A Neuropathologic Review

Laurence Edward Becker

Department of Pathology, The Hospital for Sick Children, 555 University Avenue, Toronto, Ontario M5G 1X8, Canada.

Although alternating hemiplegia of varying severity occurring in childhood has been well described from the clinical perspective (1–3), neuropathologic accounts are nonexistent. This childhood syndrome is usually accompanied by other neurologic findings, such as dystonic posturing, choreoathetoid movements, and progressive cognitive impairment (2,3). The underlying mechanism of this disorder is not understood, although complicated migraine (1,4,5), seizure activity (6,7), moyamoya disease (8,9), and mitochondrial encephalopathies (10) have all been considered. A recent report of familial alternating hemiplegia has suggested an autosomal dominant pattern of transmission based on a karyotype revealing a balanced reciprocal translocation [t(3;9) (p26;q34)] (11). One of the missing links in our understanding of this disorder is neuropathologic documentation. This chapter therefore describes the clinicopathological documentation available in a case of alternating hemiplegia and discusses its implications.

CASE REPORT

The patient, a boy, died at the age of 4 (1). He had been born after a normal pregnancy and full-term gestation. At birth, labor was prolonged and delivery was breech. His birth weight was 3,965 g. Shortly after birth, his mother noticed certain abnormalities: the child had irregular jerking movements of the eyes, constant movement of the tongue, and dry flaking skin. These disappeared by 1 month of age, and so, despite some delay in his development, the parents thought that the child was normal. From 3 months of age, the boy experienced episodes of hemiplegia involving one side or the other. These appeared to be spontaneous in onset, although they were sometimes thought to be related to excitement and frustration. They were frequently preceded by periorbital redness, crying, yawning, and scratching of the head. After about 15 minutes after the onset of an episode, the child became weak and limp, sometimes on the right side, other times on the left. This weakness developed over a period of 2–5 minutes. On occasions, the patient experienced double hemiplegia along with difficulty in swallowing and crying and later in speaking. The weakness usually resolved within 24 to 48 hours but some-times persisted for as long as 3 weeks. Interestingly, the patient's mother suffered intermittent, generalized headaches, and at age 21 had experienced an episode of right hemiplegia associated with left hemicrania, with disappearance of headaches within 2 days. She had exhibited no further neurologic symptoms. There was no family history of seizure disorder.

When the boy was admitted to hospital at 8 months of age, the results of his neurologic and physical examinations were considered normal, although develop-mentally he appeared to be at about the 6-month level. Karyotype investigation at the time showed a normal male chromosome pattern. Results of phenylketonuria testing and reducing substances in the urine were both negative, and no evidence of mucopolysaccharidosis was found. The boy's bone age was estimated to be 6 months. EEG showed minimal asymmetry that was not felt to be significant. The child was discharged with a diagnosis of minimal delayed development.

At 16 months of age, he was again admitted, this time for a hemiplegic episode. Psychomotor evaluation indicated that the child was performing tasks at the 9- to 11-month level and his intelligence quotient was estimated at 58. Results of right retrograde brachial arteriogram and EEG were both normal. He was discharged on medication that included both phenytoin and phenobarbitone.

At 20 months of age, he was admitted because of a hemiplegic episode that had occurred 48 hours earlier. On examination, he was well developed and well nourished but had an apparent right hemiparesis of mild degree. During this hospi-talization, the weakness shifted to the left side. Cerebrospinal fluid studies, arte-riography, air encephalography, and EEG all yielded normal results.

At 3½ years of age, he was admitted for reassessment of his neurologic condition and consideration for institutional care. At this time, he had been suffering 5–6 episodes per month, the most recent one (left-sided) having occurred 24 hours be-fore admission. On examination, he was considered retarded, with an IQ of 40. Physical examination revealed dystonic posturing of the limbs.

On his last admission, to an acute care hospital at the age of 4 years, examination revealed a mild left hemiparesis, and he was noted to have some dystonic posturing. In addition, he had experienced a left-sided seizure that lasted approximately 10 minutes and was terminated by intravenous Valium. The child was placed in a chronic care institution and died suddenly at the age of 4 years, 5 months. The cause of death at autopsy was established as severe bronchopneumonia secondary to aspi-ration of gastric contents.

At autopsy, the child was 100 cm in length and had a head circumference of 49.5 cm. Systemic examination results were normal apart from bronchopneumonia docu-mented in both right and left lungs. There were patchy areas of inflammatory reac-tion with polymorph infiltration, primarily in a peribronchial distribution. Aspirated gastric contents could also be identified; in some areas, the alveoli were filled with exudate. Skeletal muscle was histologically normal.

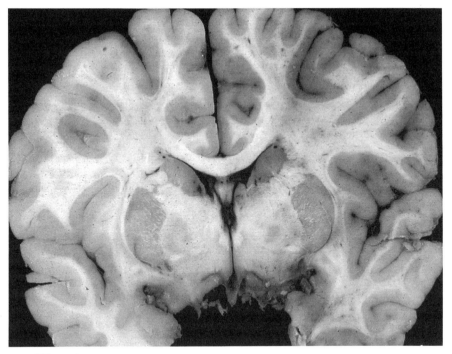

FIG. 1. Coronal section of the brain showing well-preserved gray and white matter.

NEUROPATHOLOGIC FINDINGS

The brain weighed 1,159 g. Examination of the brain after fixation showed that the cerebral hemispheres were symmetrical and the gyral patterns normal (Fig. 1). Leptomeninges were thin and delicate except for some mild congestion over the right parietal region. Examination of the circle of Willis and other vasculature revealed no gross anatomical variation from normal. Serial 1.0 cm coronal sections of the cerebral hemispheres showed that gray and white matter were clearly differentiated. The ventricles were of normal size. The caudate nucleus, putamen, globus pallidus, and thalamus were normal, although the globus pallidus was slightly darker. Transverse sections of midbrain, cerebellum, pons, medulla, and spinal cord were normal.

Extensive histologic examination of the brain was performed. Examination of the vasculature included sections of basilar artery, right carotid artery, right middle cerebral artery, right anterior cerebral artery, left carotid artery, posterior communicating artery, right posterior cerebral artery, inferior cerebellar artery, and left superior cerebellar artery. No abnormalities were noted. All sections from the following areas were stained with hematoxylin-eosin and luxol-fast blue: midbrain, pons, medulla, spinal cord, globus pallidus (right and left), thalamus (right and left) motor cortex (left), hippocampus (left and right), frontal cortex (right), calcarine cortex (right), cerebellum, cerebellar dentate nuclei, and cerebellar vermis. Some of these areas were chosen for immunohistochemical study using antiserum to glial fibrillary acidic protein (GFAP). Focal astrogliosis was present in the dorsomedial and lateral dorsal nuclei of the thalamus (Fig. 2). Extensive bilateral neuronal loss and astrogliosis were seen in the hippocampi (Fig. 3). Almost all pyramidal neurons in CA_1 and CA_3 were lost, together with many in CA_2. Residual neurons were identified within a thick network of astrogliosis throughout these areas. The dentate granular cell layer was also affected; both neuronal loss and astrogliosis were identified.

DISCUSSION

Alternating hemiplegia of childhood was first described by Verret and Steele in 1971 (1) in their account of eight patients, including the child described in this case report. On the basis of findings in these children and in those reported by others (2,3,11), the following have been suggested as diagnostic features: repeated episodes of hemiplegia, varying in severity and duration and involving either side or both sides of the body; occurrence before 18 months of age; other paroxysmal clinical signs such as dystonic posturing, choreoathetoid movements, tonic spells, and nystagmus; and progressive cognitive and neurologic deterioration.

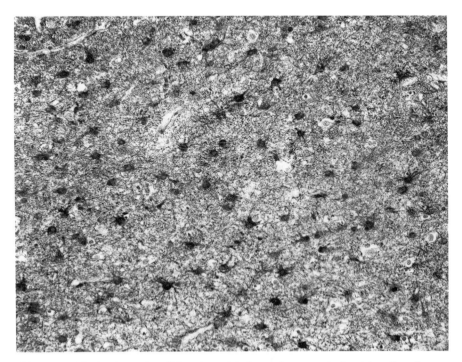

FIG. 2. Astrogliosis of dorsal medial nucleus of thalamus. Immunocytochemistry with antiserum to GFAP, × 300.

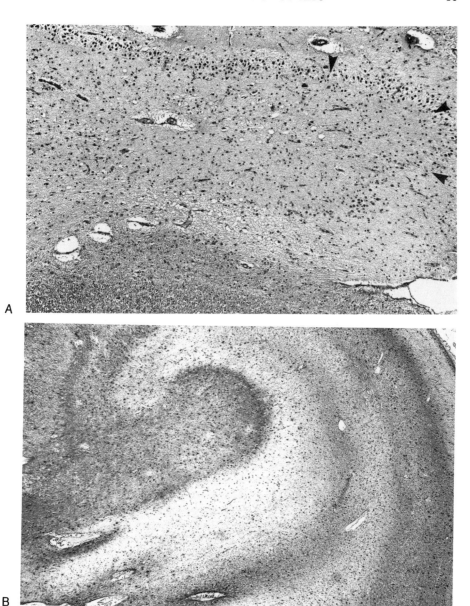

FIG. 3. A: Neuronal loss in Ammon's horn, maximum in CA_1 and CA_3. Dentate granule cell layer also shows neuronal depletion *(arrowheads)*. Hematoxylin-eosin and luxol fast blue, $\times 300$. **B:** Extensive astrogliosis throughout hippocampus. Immunocytochemistry with antiserum to GFAP, $\times 30$.

The patient described in this report had all of these features. Investigation using EEG, arteriography, and other laboratory methods ruled out arteriopathies such as moyamoya disease. Although mitochondrial encephalomyopathies would not likely have been considered 20 years ago, no lactic acidosis was noted and examination of skeletal muscle at autopsy revealed no histologic abnormalities.

The occurrence in the mother of a single episode of migraine associated with transient hemiplegia could suggest a diagnosis of complicated migraine (1). However, even though migraine is known to be rarely associated with alternating hemiplegia, dystonic posturing, choreiform movements, and cognitive decline would be distinctly unusual (4,5,11).

An epileptic syndrome could be considered in the differential diagnosis of alternating hemiplegia, but the absence of EEG changes, lack of therapeutic response to antiepileptic medication, and progressive neurologic deterioration weaken its likelihood (11).

Since the original report of eight cases (1), several clinical investigations have been conducted in subsequent cases in an effort to explain the pathogenesis of alternating hemiplegia of childhood. Studies of cerebral blood flow during and between episodes have yielded inconsistent results; an increase, decrease, and no change in blood flow have all been recorded in the hemisphere contralateral to the hemiplegia (12,13). Between hemiplegic episodes, both cerebral blood flow measured by single photon emission computerized tomography (SPECT) and cerebral metabolism as assessed by positron emission tomography (PET) were reported to be decreased (14–17). Most EEG investigations carried out during hemiplegic attacks have not shown epileptiform or consistent abnormal activity; exceptions include the report of Dalla Bernardina et al. (18), which showed focal EEG changes contralateral to the hemiplegia, and that of Hosking et al. (19), which showed diffuse nonlateralizing slow-wave abnormalities in some cases. During attacks, studies have indicated no changes in auditory brainstem evoked potentials (20), but reversible alterations of somatosensory evoked potentials have been reported (21,22).

In general, these studies have produced little or nothing in the way of consistent, positive information that would enhance our understanding of the pathophysiology of alternating hemiplegia of childhood. However, the availability of a complete neuropathologic examination creates an opportunity for further documentation of this disorder. A detailed dissection of the circle of Willis together with histologic examination of cross-sections of the major arteries showed no abnormality. The brain weight was within expected limits. Despite the cognitive decline in this child, examination of the cerebral cortex showed no atrophy and no myelination abnormalities. The most striking finding was the extensive neuronal loss and astrogliosis of the pyramidal layer of both hippocampi. Although mesial temporal sclerosis is a consistent observation in partial complex seizures, the extent and degree of neuronal loss in the hippocampus in this child was much greater than commonly seen in temporal lobe resections for seizures in patients refractory to medication. In addition, there was significant astrogliosis of the thalamus, something not seen in patients with partial complex seizures. The caudate nucleus, putamen, and globus pallidus showed no significant astrogliosis.

Damage to neurons in selected areas of the brain, shown through neuropathologic examination, elicits a vigorous astroglial response. Although the mechanism of neuronal death remains unexplained, several possibilities exist. In hypoxic-ischemic insults and in epilepsy, excitatory amino acids have been implicated in neuronal demise (23–25). Furthermore, a recent report (26) has found elevated excitatory amino acids in the plasma of migraine patients but not in that of others with tension headaches or of healthy controls. Between migrainous attacks, glutamic acid and aspartate levels were elevated and were even further increased during an episode (26). Can a relationship between the vasoconstriction phase of migraine (associated with reduced blood flow), and neuronal damage be established? Transient neurologic deficits occur more frequently with childhood migraine, and therefore severe vasospasm could produce relative ischemia with a risk of neuronal injury. Diminished oxygen delivery could lead to decreased adenosine triphosphatase (ATP) synthesis with failure of ionic pumps and cessation of ATP-dependent re-uptake of glutamate and aspartate neurotransmitters. These events could lead in turn to a prolonged stimulation of the N-methyl-D aspartate (NMDA), kainate, and quisqualate receptors (23–25). Excess sodium and calcium could then enter the neuron through the opened NMDA and other receptor channels; the result could be activation of lipases, proteins, and endonucleases, destruction of the structural integrity of the neuron, and eventual cell death (23–25).

Localization of the neuropathology in alternating hemiplegia largely to the hippocampus might be explained on the basis, first, of selective susceptibility of neurons in this region and, second, of relative resistance to the toxicity of NMDA of neurons in other regions because of the presence of the enzyme nicotinamide adenine dinucleotide phosphate (NADPH-) diaphorase (27). Identification of neurons resistant or sensitive to excitatory neurotransmitters suggests an explanation for the patterns of neuronal vulnerability that occur with hypoxic-ischemic insults. In instances where such insults (vasoconstriction) are less significant, neuronal damage may be milder and leave no permanent sequelae. However, repetitive episodes of vasoconstriction with hemiplegia of varied severity occurring at different stages of maturation could cause progressive neuronal damage.

The neuropathologic findings in the child discussed in this case report are consistent with recurrent episodes of hypoxia-ischemia. The extensive bilateral involvement of the hippocampi would explain the progressive cognitive decline. The neuronal loss and astrogliosis in Ammon's horn could also act as an epileptic focus and account for the seizures that occurred during the later clinical course. The dystonia and choreoathetoid movements are not strongly correlated with pathologic observations; the caudate and putamen were free of significant astrogliosis and the globus pallidus showed only minimal gliosis. The neuropathologic identification of astrogliosis in the thalamus is not easily correlated with clinical symptomatology.

Although the pathophysiology of alternating hemiplegia is not firmly established, an ischemic (vasoconstrictive) basis seems most consistent with the clinical and neuropathologic observations in the child described. However, alternating hemiplegia may be caused by different factors manifesting as a characteristic group of clinical signs and symptoms. As more cases become available for neuropathologic examination, the pathogenesis of this clinical syndrome will become better understood.

REFERENCES

1. Verret S, Steele JC. Alternating hemiplegia in childhood: a report of eight patients with complicated migraine beginning in infancy. *Pediatrics* 1971;47:675–680.
2. Krägeloh I, Aicardi J. Alternating hemiplegia in infants: report of five cases. *Dev Med Child Neurol* 1980;22:784–791.
3. Aicardi J. Alternating hemiplegia of childhood. *Int Fed* 1987;2:115–119.
4. Ohta M, Araki S, Kuroiwa Y. Familial occurrence of migraine with a hemiplegic syndrome and cerebellar manifestations. *Neurology* 1967;17:813–817.
5. Young GF, Leon-Barth CA, Green J. Familial hemiplegic migraine, retinal degeneration, deafness, and nystagmus. *Arch Neurol* 1970;23:201–209.
6. Lee H, Lerner A. Transient inhibitory seizures mimicking crescendo TIAs. *Neurology* 1990;40: 165–166.
7. Tinuper P, Cerullo A, Cirignotta F, Cortelli P, Lugaresi E, Montagna P. Nocturnal paroxysmal dystonia with short-lasting attacks: three cases with evidence of an epileptic frontal lobe origin of seizures. *Epilepsia* 1990;31:549–556.
8. Carlson CB, Harvey FH, Loop J. Progressive alternating hemiplegia in early childhood and basal arterial stenosis and telangiectasia (moyamoya syndrome). *Neurology* 1973;23:734–744.
9. Cornelio-Nieto JO, Davila-Gutierrez G, Ferreyro-Irigoyen R, Alcala H. Acute hemiplegia in childhood and alternating hemiconvulsions secondary to Moya-Moya disease. Report of a case associated with Down's syndrome. *Bol Med Hosp Infant Mex* 1990;47:39–42.
10. Schapira AVH. Mitochondrial disorders. *Curr Opin Neurol Neurosurg* 1990;3:425–430.
11. Mikati MA, Maguire H, Barlow CF, et al. A syndrome of autosomal dominant alternating hemiplegia: clinical presentation mimicking intractable epilepsy; chromosomal studies; and physiologic investigations. *Neurology* 1992;42:2251–2257.
12. Tada H, Miyake S, Yamada M, Iwamoto H, Morooka K, Sakuragawa N. A patient with alternating hemiplegia in childhood. *No To Hattatsu* 1989;21:283–288.
13. Nakamura Y, Nagano T, Mizuguchi M, et al. Alternating hemiplegia in infants: a single case report. *No To Hattatsu* 1986;18:406–412.
14. Zupanc ML, Dobkin JA, Perlman SB. Iodine 123 iodoamphetamine single-photon emission computed tomography brain imaging in a child with alternating hemiplegia. *Ann Neurol* 1989;26:454–455 (abst).
15. Siemes H, Casaer P. Alternating hemiplegia in childhood: Clinical report and single photon emission computed tomography study. *Monatsschr Kinderheilkd* 1988;136:467–470.
16. Kanazawa O, Shirasaka Y, Hatori H, Okuno T, Mikawa H. Ictal ^{99m}Tc-HMPAO SPECT in alternating hemiplegia. *Pediatr Neurol* 1991;7:121–124.
17. Hattori H, Hashizuka S, Matsuaka O, Murata R, Ueda T. Alternating hemiplegia in infants: a case report with abnormal findings in ABR (auditory brain stem response) and SPECT (single photon emission CT). *Jpn J Pediatr* 1989;42:77–82.
18. Dalla Bernardina B, Capovilla G, Trevisan E, et al. Alternating hemiplegia in childhood. In: Andermann F, Lugaresi E, eds. *Migraine and epilepsy.* Boston: Butterworths; 1987:188–201.
19. Hosking GP, Cavanagh NPC, Wilson J. Alternating hemiplegia: complicated migraine of infancy. *Arch Dis Child* 1978;53:656–659.
20. Santanelli P, Guerrini R, Dravet C, Genton P, Bureau M, Farnarier G. Brainstem auditory evoked potentials in alternating hemiplegia: ictal versus interictal assessment in one case. *Clin Electroencephalogr* 1990;21:51–54.
21. Imai T, Minami R, Ishikawa Y, Okabe M, Matsumoto H. Reversible changes of somatosensory-evoked potentials in a child with alternating hemiplegia [Letter]. *J Child Neurol* 1990;5:71–72.
22. Ishikawa Y, Imai T, Okabe M, et al. A case of alternating hemiplegia in infancy—ictal SSEP findings. *No To Hattatsu* 1989;21:495–497.
23. Rothman SM, Olney JW. Glutamate and the pathophysiology of hypoxic-ischemic brain damage. *Ann Neurol* 1986;19:105–111.

24. Meldrum B. Excitatory amino acids and anoxic/ischaemic brain damage. *Trends Neurosci* 1985;8: 47–48.
25. Benveniste H, Drejer J, Schousboe A, Diemer NH. Elevation of extracellular concentrations of glutamate and aspartate in rat hippocampus during transient cerebral ischemia monitored by intracerebral microdialysis. *J Neurochem* 1984;43:1369–1374.
26. Ferrari MD, Odink J, Bos KD, Malessy MJA, Bruyn GW. Neuroexcitatory plasma amino acids are elevated in migraine. *Neurology* 1990;40:1582–1586.
27. Ferriero DM, Arcavi LJ, Sagar SM, McIntosh TK, Simon RP. Selective sparing of NADPH-diaphorase neurons in neonatal hypoxia-ischemia. *Ann Neurol* 1988;24:670–676.

Alternating Hemiplegia of Childhood, edited by
Frederick Andermann, Jean Aicardi, and Federico Vigevano,
Raven Press, Ltd., New York © 1995.

7

Differential Diagnosis of Alternating Hemiplegia of Childhood

John Wilson

*Department of Neurology, Great Ormond Street Hospital for Children,
Great Ormond Street, London WCIN 3JH, England.*

Because the etiology and pathogenesis of alternating hemiplegia of childhood (AHC) are unknown, discussion of this unique syndrome inevitably overlaps with discussion of the nosology of the condition. Is it vascular, perhaps migrainous? Is it dysrhythmic, i.e., epileptic? Is it a bizarre metabolic disorder on a par with remitting-relapsing conditions such as Leigh's disease and other forms of mitochondrially-mediated lactic acidoses, hyperammonemia, Hartnup disease? But none of these latter examples really match the abrupt onset, and usually abruptly ending, sleep-mediated remission of attacks of what in some patients proves to be inexorably alternating lateralized weakness.

It is this distinctive feature which makes the differentiation from hemiplegic migraine easy in the majority of cases, although some patients with alternating hemiplegia do have characteristic migrainous symptoms, viz., photophobia, pallor, nausea, headache. In my experience these are not rare, and I suspect are coincidental phenomena. Migraine is a common disorder in childhood.

Disregarding, for the time being, the possibility that some patients with hemiplegic cerebral palsy and others with acute juvenile hemiplegia have suffered from the permanent sequelae of unusually severe attacks of hemiplegic migraine, persistent and evolving neurological deficits are not usually considered to be a feature of this condition. In AHC, by contrast, there is an evolving deficit characterized by ataxia, chorea, and mild to severe learning disability. Paroxysmal dyskinesia is an equally improbable alternative diagnosis.

In my experience the major difficulty in diagnosis arises in the first year of life when typically tonic-clonic and sometimes myoclonic attacks with corresponding EEG abnormalities mask the later evolution into alternating hemiplegia. I am aware that some deny (somewhat intemperately I fear) that epileptic phenomena ever occur in this condition. I think this is a mistaken retrospective view promulgated when the child has been seen and the correct diagnosis made long after the transition from epilepsy to hemiplegic attacks, usually in the second half of infancy.

At least two of my patients have continued to have occasional nonfocal seizures as distinct episodes separate from hemiparesis in later childhood. However, in the majority of children after the second year there is neither clinical nor electro-physiological evidence of epilepsy. Consciousness is never impaired, even on those occasions when there are bilateral attacks with consequent pseudobulbar signs.

The condition which seems to resemble most closely alternating hemiplegia as usually understood is that of autosomal dominant alternating hemiplegia reported by Mikati (see Chapter 16). I have never encountered such a family but clearly affected members have many features in common with the sporadic cases of alternating hemiplegia which form the substance of this volume. None of my patients has ever reproduced, nor is any likely to do so, and we will have to await the development of an appropriate gene probe for the Mikati disorder to know whether or not the sporadic condition represent mutations of the same malady. In the Great Ormond Street series of patients, although there was a family history of migraine in 50% of our patients, some with both parents affected, none of the parents had features of hemiplegic migraine.

In the early stages, when the episodic hemiparetic character of the disease is first recognized, other conditions such as moya-moya syndrome and microglioma have to be considered, but diagnostic imaging, especially magnetic resonance imaging and angiography should easily distinguish these conditions.

Alternating Hemiplegia of Childhood, edited by
Frederick Andermann, Jean Aicardi, and Federico Vigevano,
Raven Press, Ltd., New York © 1995.

8

A Genetic Perspective of Alternating Hemiplegia of Childhood

Eva Andermann and Frederick Andermann

*Departments of Neurology, Neurosurgery, and Pediatrics, McGill University,
Montreal Neurological Hospital and Institute, 3801 University Street,
Montreal, Quebec H3A 2B4, Canada.*

Alternating hemiplegia of childhood (AHC) in identical twins has been described by Dalla Bernardina and colleagues. The other patients with the classical form of the disorder have all been sporadic, and the main neurological features have not been present in first degree or other relatives. This would imply that the disorder is not genetically determined.

The occurrence of migraine, especially classical migraine in many, if not all pedigrees, occurring in at least one parent, most often the mother, suggests that there may be a relationship between the two disorders. Migraine with aura or classical migraine is found more often than expected by chance. At least the migraine, with its well known genetic determination may be related to the mechanism of alternating hemiplegia. This view is not, however, universally accepted, and the importance of migraine in this disorder remains a matter of debate (see Chapter 1).

In this volume it has been shown that attacks of alternating and bilateral hemiplegia are not specific for the classical disorder. Attacks which share many or most of the features may be encountered in more unusual and specific disorders. The autosomal dominant form described by Mikati (see Chapter 16) presents with attacks which, taken out of genetic context, may not be easily distinguished. Though chromosome studies in patients with the classical sporadic form have so far been normal, the finding of a translocation in the family reported by Mikati suggests that further cytogenetic studies should be performed.

Alternating hemiplegia arising exclusively out of sleep and with an apparently benign prognosis (see Chapter 17) represents another example of a genetically determined disorder. In this family, as in one originally mentioned by Verret and Steele, two siblings were affected suggesting the possibility of autosomal recessive inheritance. In our family too, there was a clear history of classical migraine, again raising the question of a relationship between these two disorders; again, however, a causal relationship could not be proven. That AHC may be related to a specific mutation is illustrated by a patient with pyruvate decarboxylase deficiency reported by Silver et al. (see Chapter 20).

One may conclude that AHC may be related to several distinct disorders. These may well have a distinct genetic determination, and a search for specific etiologies must still be undertaken. Most children presenting with alternating hemiplegia however, have the disorder as defined by Bourgeois and Aicardi (see Chapter 1), and the mechanism of this condition still eludes us. The study of this form and of related disorders has allowed us to identify an unusual negative motor disorder which has different genetic determinations that must be kept in mind in the differential diagnosis of hemiplegia, especially occurring on alternate sides in childhood.

Alternating Hemiplegia of Childhood, edited by
Frederick Andermann, Jean Aicardi, and Federico Vigevano,
Raven Press, Ltd., New York © 1995.

9

Metabolic Studies in Alternating Hemiplegia of Childhood

Raffaella Cusmai, Enrico Bertini, and *Andrea Bartuli

*Section of Neurophysiology; and *Section of Metabolic Diseases,
"Bambino Gesù" Children's Hospital; Piazza S. Onofrio, 4, 00165 Rome, Italy.*

Dystonic or tonic attacks in alternating hemiplegia of childhood (AHC) are frequently associated with or precede hemiplegic attacks. Sometimes these dystonic attacks may occur in isolation and may be present at the onset of the disease. Later in the course of the illness, many patients with AHC show ongoing dystonic posturing together with mental deficiency.

Another characteristic feature of the hemiplegic attacks is that they are reversed or aborted by sleep. This is probably the most characteristic aspect of this disorder and recently it has been suggested that sleep should be induced by pharmacological means in order to terminate the hemiplegic attacks (1).

Dystonia with marked diurnal variation or Segawa's disease is a condition that shares a similar fluctuation of neurological symptoms. Biopterin deficiency with reduced CSF concentrations of dopamine and serotonin metabolites, namely homovanillic (HVA) and 5-hydroxyindoleacetic acid (5-HIAA), has been reported in two adult patients and three children with dystonia with marked diurnal variation (2), and in a patient with dihydrobiopterin synthesis defect (3) in whom symptoms clearly improved after sleep. Other authors observed reduced levels of CSF biopterins in patients with generalized or focal, diurnally variable, or diurnally constant dystonia (4).

Tetrahydrobiopterin (BH4), the fully reduced form of biopterin is an essential cofactor for tyrosine hydroxylase, the rate limiting enzyme of catecholamine and serotonin synthesis.

BH4 is synthesized from guanosine triphosphate through dihydrobiopterin (BH2) in several enzymatic steps (5).

Intermittent dystonia has also been described in a patient with Hartnup disease (HD) (6) who had decreased levels of CSF 5-HIAA. In HD there is a defect in renal and intestinal transport of monoamino-monocarboxylic acids. Serum levels of many amino acids are decreased, particularly tryptophan, the precursor of serotonin. It appears that HD is mainly asymptomatic unless the patient is inadequately

TABLE 1. *Metabolic studies in AHC*

Patient no.	Sex	Age	Onset	5-HIAA	HVA	HMPG	Neopterin	Biopterin	%B	Phe	Tyr
1	F	2 yrs 11 mos	16 mos	110	612	45	11	22	67	18	12
2	M	5 yrs 1 mos	15 days	124	622	np	15	36	70	18	12
3	F	5 yrs 4 mos	15 days	109	495	48	11	37	77	20	16
4	M[a]	5 yrs 4 mos	9 mos	138	486	51	10.8	29	73	np	np
Normal values				>80	>250	56 ± 9[b]	9–20	10–30		<20	<25

[a]In this case investigations were performed during an attack of AHC.
HVA, homovanillic acid (nmol/l); 5-HIAA, 5-hydroxy indoleacetic acid (nmol/l); HMPG, hydroxymethoxyphenylglycol (nmol/l); neopterin and biopterin are given in mmol/mol creatinine; %B, ratio of neopterin to biopterin; Phe, phenylalanine (μmol/l); Tyr, tyrosine (μmol/l); np, not performed.
[b]Lekman A, et al. *Clin Genet* 1990;37:173–178.

nourished. Thus, these data show that a disorder of dopamine and serotonin may be an important pathogenetic factor in fluctuating dystonia.

In AHC, hemiplegic attacks are frequently provoked by emotion or sudden stress. This clinical feature suggests a similarity to cataplexy, where abrupt and reversible decrease or loss of muscle tone involves the entire voluntary musculature. Cataplectic attacks, however, do not involve ocular movement and do not last more than 30 minutes. The neurochemistry of cataplexy is not fully elucidated but animal studies suggest that catecholamine systems play an important role in canine narcolepsy-cataplexy. CSF dopamine has been found to be decreased in patients with narcolepsy (7).

The aim of this study was to find a biochemical marker in AHC, considering the analogy of symptoms with other disorders that share similar clinical features.

We screened four patients, 2 boys and 2 girls, with AHC for intermediate metabolism and biopterins as well as catecholamines in CSF.

The patients were between 2 years 11 months and 5 years 4 months old; onset of symptoms appeared between 15 days and 16 months of life. Investigations were performed between 1 year 7 months and 5 years 3 months after onset of the disease. In patient 4, laboratory studies were performed during an attack of AHC (Table 1).

Each patient had the following investigations: routine hematological studies, serum and CSF lactate, serum ammonia, urinary and CSF amino acids, urinary organic acids, urinary and CSF biopterins, CSF HVA (homovanillic acid), 5-HIAA (5-hydroxyindoleacetic acid), and HMPG (hydroxymethoxyphenylglycol).

Amino acids were measured by amino-analyzer; urinary organic acids were measured by gas chromatography and mass spectroscopy; CSF pterin studies were assessed by high-performance liquid chromatography.

Hematologic exams, serum and CSF lactate and amino acids, urinary amino acids and organic acids were normal. Values for biopterins, HVA, 5–HIAA, and HMPG were in the normal range for age and are summarized in Table 1.

The present study did not show any abnormality of intermediate metabolism or of biogenic amine metabolism in AHC. Pathogenesis of the disorder remains to be fully elucidated.

ACKNOWLEDGMENTS

We would like to thank Dr. N. Blau of the University Children's Hospital, Zurich, Switzerland and the Department of Psychiatry and Neurochemistry of Gothenburg University, Sweden for the study of biogenic amines in CSF.

REFERENCES

1. Siemes H. Rectal Chloral Hydrate for Alternating Hemiplegia of Childhood. *Dev Med Child Neurol* 1990;32:931.
2. Fink JK, Barton N, Cohen W, Lowenberg W, Burns RS, Hallett M. Dystonia with marked diurnal variation associated with biopterin deficiency. *Neurology* 1988;38:707–711.

3. Tanaka K, Yoneda M, Nakagima T, Miyatake T, Owada M. Dihydrobiopterin synthesis defect: an adult with diurnal fluctuation of symptoms. *Neurology* 1987;37:519–522.
4. Le Witt PA, Miller LP, Levine RA, Lowenberg W, Neuman RP, Papavasiliou A, Rayes A, Eldridge R, Burns S. Tetrahydrobiopterin in dystonia: Identification of abnormal metabolism and therapeutic trials. *Neurology* 1986:36:760–764.
5. Curtius HC, Blau N, Kuster T. Pterins. In: Hommes FA, ed. *Techniques in diagnostic human biochemical genetics: a laboratory manual.* New York: Wiley-Liss, 1991;377–396.
6. Darras BT, Ampola MG, Dietz WH, Gilmore HE. Intermittent dystonia in Hartnup disease. *Pediatr Neurol* 1989;5:118–120.
7. Montplaisir J, DeChamplain J, Young SN, Missala K, Sourkes TL, Walsh J, Remillard G. Narcolepsy and idiopatic hypersomnia: biogenic amines and related compounds in CSF. *Neurology* 1982; 32:1299–1302.

Alternating Hemiplegia of Childhood, edited by
Frederick Andermann, Jean Aicardi, and Federico Vigevano,
Raven Press, Ltd., New York © 1995.

10

Alternating Hemiplegia of Childhood: Epilepsy and Electroencephalographic Investigations

Bernardo Dalla Bernardina, Elena Fontana, Vito Colamaria,
Emanuele Zullini, Francesca Darra, Licia Giardina, Anna Franco,
and Alessandra Montagnini

Cattedra di Neuropsichiatria Infantile, Policlinico Borgo Roma, 37134 Verona, Italy.

Alternating hemiplegia of childhood (AHC) is a peculiar disorder rarely reported in the literature and little known in clinical practice. The etiology and pathogenesis are much debated, particularly regarding its relationship to basilar migraine. A clinical and polygraphic analysis of eight patients allows us to more appropriately delineate the electroclinical features of the syndrome and to contribute further information to the discussion concerning the relationship between AHC and epilepsy.

CLINICAL FEATURES

Our study concerns eight personal cases (including two monozygotic twins) longitudinally followed at the Child Neuropsychiatric Service of the University of Verona; the initial histories of patients 1, 2, and 3 have previously been reported by Dalla Bernardina et al. (1).

We studied five females and three males, a family history of migraine being present in three of the patients. Familial antecedents for epilepsy were absent and psychomotor development at onset was normal in half the patients, abnormal in the others. Hemiplegic episodes had their peak of onset between 1 and 5 months (range 15 days to 18 months) and epileptic seizures, present in four children, appeared toward the end of the first year of life (9 to 14 months). The mean age at the last follow-up was 13 years (range 4.5 to 20 years) (Table 2).

As shown in Table 2, psychomotor development was more or less severely impaired in all but one patient. Dystonia and choreoathetosis were prominent neurological signs; although present in all patients, they were particularly severe in three. Pyramidal tract signs were present in four individuals. Two children were severely

TABLE 1. *Clinical features of patients with AHC*

Patient	Sex	Development before first attack	Age at first attack	Familial antecedents for migraine	Familial antecedents for epilepsy	Epileptic seizures (age of onset)
1[a]	F	Abnormal	4 mo	—	—	11 mos
2[a]	F	Abnormal	5 mos	—	—	10 mos
3	F	Normal	3 mos	—	—	—
4	F	Normal	20 days	+	—	—
5	M	Abnormal	15 days	+	—	9 mos
6	M	Abnormal	45 days	+	—	—
7	M	Normal	18 mos	—	—	—
8	F	Normal	3 mos	—	—	14 mos

[a]Patients 1 and 2 are monozygotic twins.

retarded at the onset and never acquired speech; four had mild mental retardation, which did not worsen with age. Two children were intellectually normal.

In all cases (Table 3) the first paroxysmal manifestation consisted of a hemiplegic attack following a generally brief dystonic episode. In the majority of children, the dystonic event was accompanied by crying or other manifestations of pain, hyperpnea, various signs of autonomic disturbance, and unilateral nystagmus. These peculiar bouts of unilateral nystagmus coincided with the onset of dystonic episodes and persisted for a few minutes after the onset of the hemiplegic attack.

The hemiplegia was flaccid but deep tendon reflexes were present; however, in most cases the degree of hypotonia fluctuated because of the recurrence of dystonia during the hemiplegic attack.

The duration of a hemiplegic attack during early childhood varied from 30 minutes to several days.

Frequently, during the more prolonged attacks, the hemiplegia involved the opposite side as well, becoming a severe tetraplegia accompanied by dyspnea, drooling, and difficulty in swallowing.

The initial frequency of attacks was generally high with weekly recurrences in five children and monthly attacks in three.

Immediate precipitating factors for hemiplegia, such as emotional stress, fear, exposure to cold, sleep deprivation, and prolonged crying were documented in six patients.

Documented factors leading to recovery were rest and sleep; however, following very brief sleep, hemiplegia reappeared a few minutes after awaking. Rectal diazepam led to cessation of attacks in three subjects but the effect was transient when the period of sleep was brief.

Severity, duration, and frequency of the attacks progressively decreased with age; at the last follow-up (Table 2) the hemiplegic attacks had stopped in four children and were rare in the other four.

All patients were treated with 5 to 10 mg of flunarizine daily; in three the treatment was started at the onset, and in the others after a period of evolution varying

TABLE 2. *Clinical features of patients with AHC*

Patient no.	Present age (years)	Psychomotor development	Clinical course								
			Dystonia and choreoathetosis		Pyramidal signs	Mental retardation		Hemiplegic attacks	Seizures	Episodic headaches
			Severe	Mild		Severe	Mild			
1	14	Delayed +	+		+	+		Stopped 10 years	Frequent	Yes
2	14	Delayed +	+		+	+		Stopped 10 years	Frequent	Yes
3	15	Delayed		+			+	Stopped 9 years		
4	20	Delayed		+				Stopped 12 years		Yes
5	8.5	Delayed		+	+		+	Rare	Rare	
6	19	Delayed	+		+		+	Rare		Yes
7	4.5	Normal		+				Rare		
8	10	Delayed					+	Rare	Rare	

EEG IN AHC

TABLE 3. *Frequency and duration of episodic manifestations in AHC*

Hemiplegia	8/8
Bilateral episodes with difficulty swallowing, drooling	6/8
Dystonic attacks	8/8
Pain	7/8
Unilateral nystagmus	7/8
Autonomic disturbances	6/8
Duration	30 sec to several days
Initial frequency	Several/wk : 5 several/mo : 3

from 2 to 10 years. Following treatment, the frequency of the attacks remained unchanged whereas their duration and severity was reduced in four children.

In two children whose hemiplegic attacks were invariably induced by fear, significant improvement was obtained by the addition of diazepam.

In four subjects (Table 2) recurrent migraine attacks appeared; in two they occurred following a brief and painful dystonic fit involving the face.

Four of the eight children (Table 1) had repeated epileptic seizures in addition to the hemiplegic attacks; these were long-lasting partial seizures with occipital symptomatology sometimes followed by a hemiclonic seizure. These attacks evolved to partial status epilepticus which could frequently only be stopped by intravenous or rectal diazepam and in some cases by intramuscular phenobarbital. The seizures, which occurred independently of the hemiplegic attacks, remained refractory to different antiepileptic drugs and to flunarizine over the years (Table 2).

All subjects had cranial CI scans and five had MRIs. Mild subcortical atrophy was present in two subjects, whereas the scans of the others were normal.

EEG FEATURES

Multiple EEG and polygraphic examinations during wakefulness and sleep permitted the recording of several hemiplegic attacks (Table 4) in all the children and of epileptic seizures in four.

Interictal tracings were normal both during wakefulness and sleep in five children (Figs. 1 and 7) whereas in three the background activity was slow for age and reacted poorly, with depression of posterior rhythmic activity contralateral to the hemiplegia.

Interictal epileptogenic abnormalities were never observed during wakefulness nor during sleep.

In three children no abnormalities were observed during hemiplegic attacks. In four, unilateral slowing (Figs. 1–3) was repeatedly observed during a hemiplegic attack, even when the weakness was bilateral. This slowing decreased progressively during sleep but, like the hemiplegia, reappeared a few minutes after awakening (Figs. 1–6).

One child, suffering from bilateral attacks often elicited by sudden fear, showed

TABLE 4. *EEG recordings in AHC patients*

EEG recordings					
	Patients		Patients		Patients
Interictal tracings	8	Hemiplegic attacks recorded	8	Epileptic seizures	4
Background slowing	3	Unilateral slowing	4	Parieto-occipital S-W discharges	4
Normal	5	Bilateral slowing	1		
Paroxysmal abnormalities	0	Normal during attacks	3		

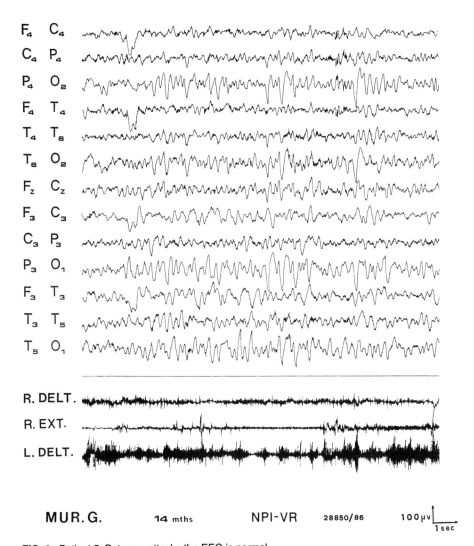

MUR. G.   **14** mths   NPI-VR   28850/86   100 μv ⌐
                                                    └─→
                                                    1 sec

FIG. 1. Patient 5. Between attacks the EEG is normal.

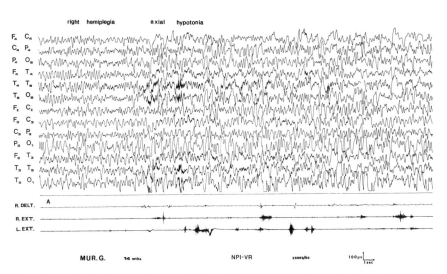

FIG. 2. Patient 5. During an attack of right hemiplegia, there is diffuse slowing predominating over the posterior regions of the left hemisphere. Note the absence of muscle activity in the EMG from the right deltoid.

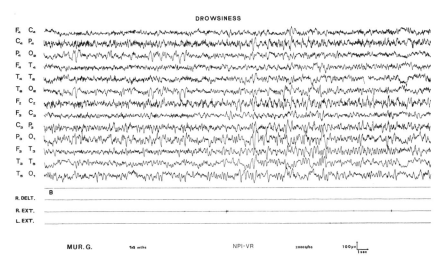

FIG. 3. Patient 5. During drowsiness the asymmetry persists. Note the predominance of slow waves over the left temporo-occipital region and that the fast, pharmacologically induced activity, is less obvious over that area.

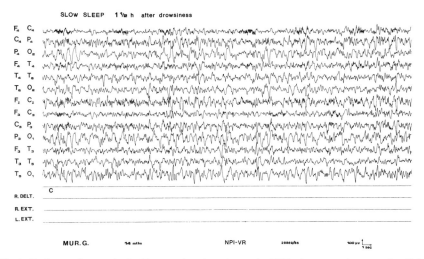

FIG. 4. Patient 5. One and a half hours after drowsiness the EEG shows persistence of a slight asymmetry with less evidence of spindle activity over the left hemisphere.

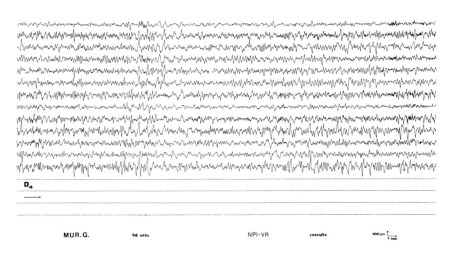

FIG. 5. Patient 5. During phase II of the second cycle, the asymmetry has disappeared. Bilateral spindles are present.

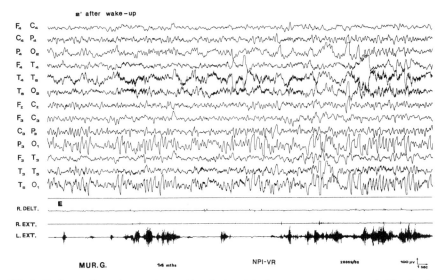

FIG. 6. Patient 5. Two minutes after waking the hemiplegia reappears, accompanied by slowing over the posterior regions of the left hemisphere. (Note the absence of muscular activity on the EMG from the right deltoid and extensor.)

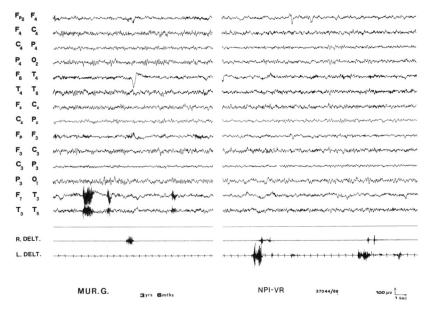

FIG. 7. Patient 5. The same child at the age of three years six months. The EEG remains normal between hemiplegic attacks.

severe generalized slowing during the episodes. In this patient, sleep induced rapid improvement, but the typical pattern of paradoxical arousal consisting of slow wave activity was easily elicited during all phases of the first cycle of sleep.

The severity of the slowing tended to decrease with age in any given subject (Fig. 8); it appeared to be related more to the severity of the hemiplegia than to its duration.

Epileptic ictal events were recorded several times in two children (patients 1 and 2), three times in another (patient 5), and twice in a fourth (patient 8). In most cases the attacks were long-lasting partial seizures with initial eye deviation, loss of contact, followed by stupor with no other focal manifestations. Sometimes the seizures were accompanied by repeated gagging, often stopped only by the administration of intravenous diazepam.

The ictal EEG showed high amplitude, 2 to 2.5 Hz spike and wave activity involving the temporo-occipital regions of one hemisphere (Figs. 9 A and B and 10) or of both hemispheres alternately.

In spite of the nonepileptic nature of the hemiplegic attacks, associated epileptic seizures occurred in nearly half the cases. Ictal EEG and polygraphic recordings confirmed the focal nature of the seizures and confirmed that these were unrelated to the hemiplegic attacks.

Frequently the seizures were followed by pronounced postictal slowing over posterior head regions (Fig. 11).

In some patients unilateral, focal, myoclonic jerks occurred during the seizures concomitant with the spread of spike-wave discharges to the rolandic region. In none of the patients was a unilateral ictal or postictal deficit observed.

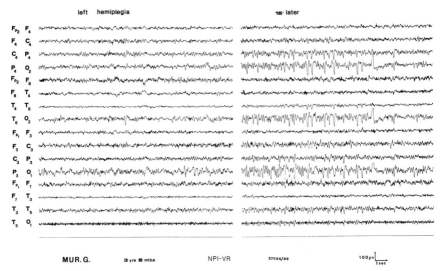

FIG. 8. Patient 5. During a left hemiplegic attack slight EEG slowing appears and disappears after a few minutes.

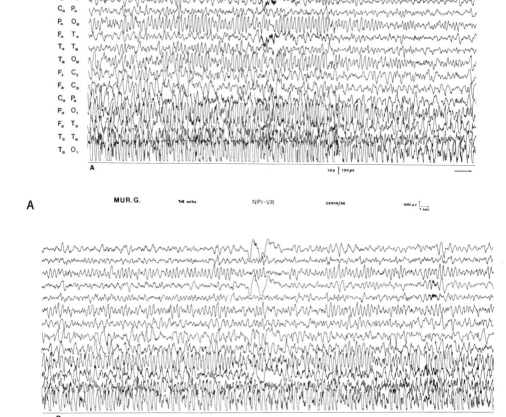

A

B

FIG. 9. A, B: Patient 5. The child has a partial seizure lasting 10 seconds characterized by loss of contact and eyes deviated to the left. Note the paroxysmal sequence of spike and polyspike and waves involving the left temporo-occipital region.

An epileptic seizure was never observed during or following a hemiplegic attack, nor did a hemiplegic attack ever follow an epileptic seizure.

DISCUSSION

The clinical features and course of our eight patients was consistent with the diagnosis of typical AHC (1–4).

The etiology of the condition remains unknown and is still the subject of ongoing debate.

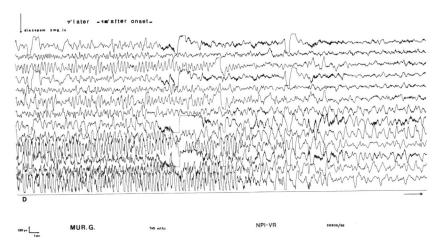

FIG. 10. Patient 5. An intravenous injection of diazepam stops the seizure. Note the significant unilateral postictal slowing in the absence of motor deficit.

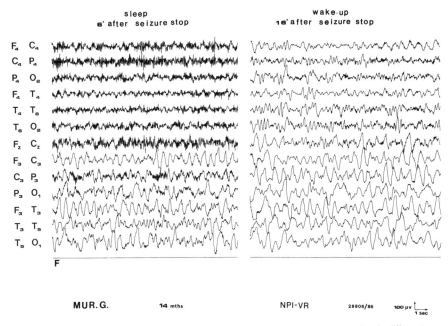

FIG. 11. Patient 5. Note the persistence of significant postictal asymmetry completely different from the slowing observed during hemiplegic attacks.

Aicardi (2) showed that the attacks of alternating hemiplegia are distinct and not epileptic in nature. Many authors (1,4–12) have recorded hemiplegic attacks without ever detecting epileptic discharge. Only Shirasaka et al. (13) published an ictal recording evoking an epileptic seizure; however, in that case, one could not be certain whether the recorded event was or was not a typical attack of alternating hemiplegia.

There are many reports (6–9, 14–16) of recurrence of epileptic seizures in patients suffering from alternating hemiplegia. Sakuragawa (3) reports a 59% incidence of epileptic seizures in Japanese patients and there is a 47% incidence in published European cases. Silver and Andermann (4) found epileptic seizures in half their patients and this has been our experience as well.

Our electroclinical study allows us to definitively confirm the previously suggested hypothesis (5) that epileptic seizures occurring in patients with AHC are quite different, from an electroclinical point of view, from hemiplegic attacks and that they have no direct connection with them.

Our data also confirm the fact that there is no specific EEG pattern that characterizes the hemiplegic attacks. In fact, as reported by most authors, during the attack the EEG can remain unchanged or show more or less significant unilateral slowing which decreases during sleep. The severity of this slowing is independent of the duration of the attack; it is, however, more evident during more severe attacks and tends to decrease with age.

CONCLUSIONS

AHC is an unusual disorder of unknown etiology, characterized by easily recognizable clinical features. The ictal EEG polygraphic recordings allow us to exclude an epileptic mechanism. Only variable, mainly unilateral slowing is found and this has no specific significance. In spite of the nonepileptic nature of the hemiplegic attacks, associated epileptic seizures occur in half the patients. Ictal EEG polygraphic recordings confirm the partial nature of the seizures and show that they are unrelated to the hemiplegic attacks.

Because of the association within the same subject, in some instances recording of paroxysmal events may be required in order to provide clarification and allow appropriate treatment.

REFERENCES

1. Krägeloh I, Aicardi J. Alternating hemiplegia in infants: report of five cases. *Dev Med Child Neurol* 1980;22:784–91.
2. Aicardi J. Alternating hemiplegia of childhood. *Int Pediatr* 1987;2;115–119.
3. Sakuragawa N. Alternating hemiplegia in childhood: 23 cases in Japan. *Brain Dev* 1992;14:283–1288.
4. Silver K, Andermann F. Alternating hemiplegia of childhood. *Neurology* 1993;43:36–41.

5. Dalla Bernardina B, Capovilla G, Trevisan E, et al. Alternating hemiplegia in childhood. In: Andermann F, Lugaresi E, eds. Migraine and epilepsy. London: Butterworths; 1987;189–201.
6. Verret S, Steele JC. Alternating hemiplegia in childhood: a report of 8 patients with complicated migraine beginning in infancy. *Pediatrics* 1971;47:675–80.
7. Hosking GP, Cavanagh NPC, Wilson J. Alternating hemiplegia: complicated migraine of infancy. *Arch Dis Child* 1978;53:656–659.
8. Zupanc ML, Dobkin JA, Perlman SB. ^{123}I-iodoamphetamine SPECT brain imaging in alternating hemiplegia. *Pediatr Neurol* 1991;7:35–38.
9. Mikati MA, Maguire H, Barlow CF, et al. A syndrome of autosomal dominant alternating hemiplegia: clinical presentation mimicking intractable epilepsy; chromosomal studies; and physiologic investigations. *Neurology* 1992;42:2251–2257.
10. Fusco L, Di Capua M, Granata T, et al. Video-EEG aspects of alternating hemiplegia. In: Gallai V, Guidetti V, eds. Juvenile headache. Elsevier Science; 1991:361–362.
11. Kanazawa O, Shirasaka Y, Hattori H, et al. Ictal ^{99m}Tc-HMPAO SPECT in alternating hemiplegia. *Pediatr Neurol* 1991;7:121–24.
12. Aminian A, Strashun A, Rose A. Alternating hemiplegia of childhood: studies of regional cerebral blood flow using ^{99m}Tc-hexamethylpropylene amine oxime single-photon emission computed tomography. *Ann Neurol* 1993;33(1):43–47.
13. Shirasaka Y, Ito M, Okuno T, Mikawa H, Yamori Y. Epileptic seizures difficult to differentiate from alternating hemiplegia in infants: a case report. *Brain Dev* 1990;12:521–524.
14. Golden GS, French JH. Basilar artery migraine in young children. *Pediatrics* 1975;56:722–726.
15. Dittrich J, Havlóva M, Nevšímalóva S. Paroxysmal hemiparesis in childhood. *Dev Med Child Neurol* 1979;21:800–807.
16. Hockaday JM. Basilar artery migraine in childhood. *Dev Med Child Neurol* 1979;21:455–463.

Alternating Hemiplegia of Childhood, edited by
Frederick Andermann, Jean Aicardi, and Federico Vigevano,
Raven Press, Ltd., New York © 1995.

11

Evoked Potentials and Blink Reflex Studies in Alternating Hemiplegia of Childhood

Matteo Di Capua and Enrico Bertini

*Section of Neurophysiology, "Bambino Gesù" Children's Hospital;
Piazza S. Onofrio, 4, 00165 Rome, Italy.*

Except for EEGs, patients with alternating hemiplegia of childhood (AHC) have not been studied extensively from a neurophysiological point of view. Only a few children have had evoked potentials recorded.

Hosking and coworkers in 1978 (1) first reported a patient studied by visual evoked potentials recorded during an attack of hemiparetic weakness. They observed a lowering of the amplitude of the cortical response. Dalla Bernardina et al. (2) then studied two children with brainstem auditory evoked potentials (BAEPs) and visual evoked potentials (VEPs) during the interictal phase, and obtained normal results. Santanelli et al. (3) studied a patient with AHC using BAEPs both during the ictal and the interictal phases, but did not find any significant difference between the two stages. Recently Imai and coworkers (4) recorded somatosensory evoked potentials (SEPs) in a 4-year-old girl. They stimulated the left median nerve at the wrist during an attack of double hemiplegia at 5 minutes as well as 30 minutes after intravenous diazepam injection, which led to cessation of the attack. The primary cortical evoked response was not clearly represented during the ictal phase. It then progressively increased in amplitude and shortened in latency following the diazepam injection.

METHODS AND RESULTS

Between January 1987 and January 1992 we performed evoked potential studies in four children with AHC, three males and one female, ranging in age from 9 months to 5 years (median age 28 months).

Brainstem auditory evoked potentials were performed in all patients; somatosensory evoked potentials, by stimulation of the median nerve at the wrist in three patients; flash visual evoked potentials in one patient; and motor evoked potentials using magnetic transcranial stimulation in two patients. All these examinations were performed during and between attacks of hemiplegia. All the results fell within normal limits (Table 1). Figure 1 shows the SEPs in patient 4. The N20 wave, that is generated from the primary cortex, did not change in latency during the ictal and the interictal states.

We also performed blink reflex studies in two patients. In both patients a normal R1 response and a delayed R2 response, both ipsilateral (R2) and contralateral (R2') to the side of stimulation were recorded. These results were obtained by stimulation of both the right and the left supraorbital nerves. Abnormalities were present during attacks of double hemiplegia, as well as in between episodes (Fig. 2).

DISCUSSION

The R1 response of the blink reflex is relayed through an oligosynaptic arc involving the pons while the R2 and R2' responses are relayed through a polysynaptic arc involving the pons and the lateral medulla (5).

A normal R1 response and a significantly delayed R2 and R2' were reported in lesions affecting the lateral medulla, as well as in patients with Wallenberg's syndrome (5). In our two patients significantly delayed R2 responses were found both during and between attacks, suggesting persistent abnormalities of the brainstem.

Normal BAEPs could be explained by the different pathways involved and by the low sensitivity of these potentials to become abnormal in pathological states which do not directly involve their generators (6). Blink reflex R2 responses, on the other hand, are involved not only in lesions directly affecting the reflex pathways, but also by lesions indirectly modifying the excitability of the polysynaptic arc (7).

In conclusion, our data using multimodal evoked potential studies exclude involvement of their different generators during attacks of AHC. Persistent abnormalities of the blink reflex, both during and between attacks, support the hypothesis of a permanent brainstem dysfunction in AHC.

TABLE 1. *Neurophysiological findings in AHC*

Patient no., sex, age (mos)	EEG	BAEPs	SEPs	VEPs	MEPs	Blink reflex
1, M, 9	NS	N	N	N	nd	+
2, F, 24	NS	N	N	nd	N	+
3, M, 20	NS	N	nd	nd	nd	nd
4, M, 60	NS	N	N	nd	N	nd

N, normal; nd, not done; NS, no specific abnormalities; +, abnormal.

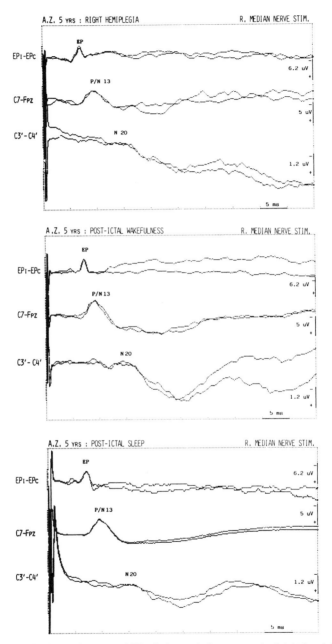

FIG. 1. Patient 4. Right median nerve SEPs during and after an attack of right hemiplegia showing normal responses from Erb's point (EP), from the neck (P/N13), and from the left sensory cortex (N20). Note that the N20 wave does not change in latency during and between attacks, EPi and EPc are Erb's point ipsilateral and contralateral to stimulation, respectively. C7 refers to cervical spine at C7. C3′ and C4′ are 2 cm behind the 10–20 International System electrode positions C3 and C4.

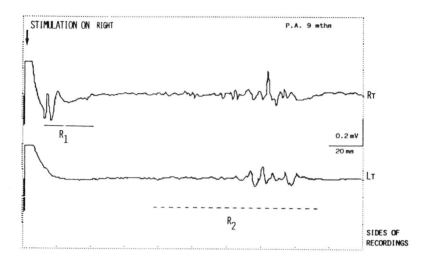

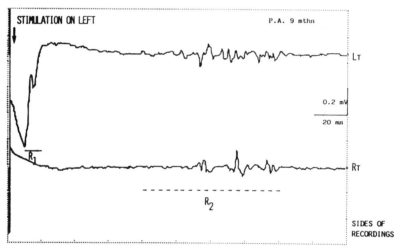

FIG. 2. Patient 1. Blink reflex during the interictal state. R1 is normal bilaterally, while a delayed R2 is evident when stimulating the supraorbital nerves, both ipsilaterally and contralaterally.

REFERENCES

1. Hosking GP, Cavanagh NPC, Wilson J. Alternating hemiplegia: complicated migraine of infancy. *Arch Dis Child* 1978;53:656–659.
2. Dalla Bernardina B, Capovilla G, Trevisan E, et al. Alternating hemiplegia in childhood. In: Andermann F, Lugaresi E, eds. *Migraine and epilepsy*. Boston: Butterworths; 1987:189–201.
3. Santanelli P, Guerrini R, Dravet C, Genton P, Bureau M, Farnarier G. Brainstem auditory evoked potentials in alternating hemiplegia: ictal vs interictal assessment in one case. *Clin Electroencephalogr* 1990;21:551–554.
4. Imai T, Okobe M, Matsumoto H. Reversible changes of somato-sensory evoked potentials in a child with alternating hemiplegia. *J Child Neurol* 1990;5:71–72.
5. Kimura J. The blink reflex. In: Kimura J, ed. *Electrodiagnosis in disease of nerve and muscle: principles and practice*. Philadelphia: Davis; 1983:323–351.
6. Chiappa KH. Brainstem anditory evoked potentials: interpretation. In Chiappa KH, ed. *Evoked potentials in clinical medicine*. New York: Raven Press; 1990:223–284.
7. Kimura J. The blink reflex as a test for brain-stem and higher central nervous system functions. In: Desmedt JE, ed. *New developments in electromyography and clinical neurophysiology*. Basel: Karger; 1973:682–691.

Alternating Hemiplegia of Childhood, edited by
Frederick Andermann, Jean Aicardi, and Federico Vigevano,
Raven Press, Ltd., New York © 1995.

12

Sleep Studies of Children with Alternating Hemiplegia of Childhood

Stefano Ricci

*Section of Neurophysiology, "Bambino Gesù" Children's Hospital,
Piazza S. Onofrio, 4, 00165 Rome, Italy.*

Attacks of alternating hemiplegia of childhood (AHC) are closely related to sleep. Their duration varies from minutes to days, and they usually cease with sleep (1). Moreover, in some patients, sleep induction by chloral hydrate is an effective therapy to stop bilateral attacks of long duration (2).

AHC is characterized by uni- or bilateral attacks of weakness, which can be provoked by stress and emotion. These clinical features are common in cataplectic attacks, which are characteristic of the adult narcoleptic syndrome (3).

The aims of our study were to record attacks of AHC during long-term EEG monitoring, including preictal EEG and postictal sleep, and to study the sleep architecture in order to evaluate possible similarities between AHC and the narcolepsy-cataplexy syndrome.

PATIENTS AND METHODS

Four children with AHC were studied, ranging in age from 10 months to 5 years 4 months. Recordings were obtained with a long-term ambulatory cassette EEG (Micromed Brain-Spy CH 24). Ten collodion electrodes were placed on the scalp, according to the 10–20 International System; horizontal electro-oculogram was also obtained. Duration of recordings ranged from 48 to 72 hours.

Ambulatory EEGs were recorded in two children during hospitalization; in the others these were performed at home.

Sleep architecture was identified by using both EEG-EOG (4) and audio signal (5).

RESULTS

Two attacks were recorded in two children. The episodes had a duration of 30 minutes in one child and of 55 minutes in the other. Clinically, they were characterized by bilateral hypotonia mixed with hypertonia and unilateral mydriasis in the first child and by right-sided hypotonia in the other. No EEG changes were observed before, during, and after the attacks. In the second child (Fig. 1) the attack stopped during sleep.

The EEG was normal in all the children except one, who presented slow and sharp waves over the right occipital area, both during wakefulness and sleep.

Sleep architecture showed no relevant abnormalities (Table 1). First REM latency, REM and slow-wave sleep percentages, sleep duration, and cycle length showed normal values when compared with age-matched children. Only in the youngest and most severely affected child did we observe frequent awakenings and excessive sleep fragmentation.

Three children among the four presented long duration sleep spindles in NREM sleep. In one we observed bilateral "extreme spindles," characterized by long duration (10 to 30 seconds) high-amplitude 10 to 12 Hz activity, recurring in a periodic fashion during stages II and III.

DISCUSSION

Our data confirm the lack of specificity of EEG patterns in AHC. Ictal and interictal EEG patterns in patients with AHC include diffuse or focal slowing over the

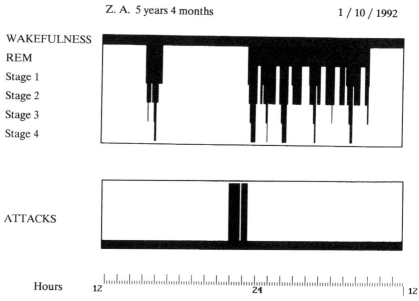

FIG. 1. Sleep-wake histogram **(Top)** of a 5-year-old boy. Two attacks, separated by a free interval of 5 minutes, were recorded **(Bottom)**. The second attack was followed by sleep. On morning awakening the child was well. Sleep architecture was normal with 60- to 90-minute cycles and a normal amount of REM sleep.

TABLE 1. Sleep architecture in AHC

Patient	Age	Day	TST	TREM	TSW	TWT	TA
AP	10 mos	1	683	33	214	756	17
		2	573	72	225	866	13
TA	2 yrs	1	693	162	114	746	4
		2	806	177	89	633	7
		3	611	198	143	828	1
PG	5 yrs	1	563	105	141	876	—
		2	561	96	129	878	—
		3	608	114	130	831	—
ZA	5 yrs	1	656	132	114	783	3
		2	660	165	116	780	2

TST, total amount of sleep time; TREM, total amount of REM sleep; TSW, total amount of slow wave sleep; TWT, total amount of wakefulness; TA, transient awakenings.

hemisphere contralateral to clinical signs (6), or nonspecific irregularities. In our series only two attacks were recorded. These were not accompanied by EEG slowing or asymmetry. No EEG abnormalities were observed before and after attacks. A single attack stopped during sleep. Subsequent sleep revealed no abnormalities, and sleep structure remained normal.

One patient had focal slow waves and spikes. Perhaps these represented postictal changes following an attack. This, however, remains uncertain, since we did not record attacks in this patient.

In three of the children we observed prolonged sleep spindles. In one, these had the characteristics of "extreme spindles." This is an unusual, though nonspecific pattern, found in 0.05% of normal children, and often related to mental retardation and/or cerebral palsy (7).

Sleep structure, sleep duration, cycle length, REM latency, and REM and slow wave sleep percentages were normal in all children. Despite the clinical evidence of a relationship between AHC attacks and sleep, the basic sleep generation processes did not seem to be abnormal in this disease.

REFERENCES

1. Aicardi J. Alternating hemiplegia of childhood. *Int Pediatr* 1987;2:115–119.
2. Siemes H. Rectal chloral hydrate for alternating hemiplegia of childhood. *Dev Med Child Neurol* 1990;32:931.
3. Kales A, Cadieux RJ, Soldatos CR, Bixler EO, Schweitzer PK, Prey WT, Vela-Bueno A. Narcolepsy-cataplexy. I. Clinical and electrophysiologic characteristics. *Arch Neurol* 1982;39:164–168.
4. Carskadon MA, Rechtschaffen A. Monitoring and staging human sleep. In: Kryger MH, Roth T, Dement WC, eds. *Principles and practice of sleep medicine*. Philadelphia: Saunders; 1989:665–683.
5. Erwin CW, Ebersole JS. Data reduction of cassette-recorded polysomnographic measures. In: Ebersole JS, ed. *Ambulatory EEG monitoring*. New York: Raven Press; 1989:257–266.
6. Dalla Bernardina B, Capovilla G, Trevisan E, et al. Alternating hemiplegia in childhood. In: Andermann F, Lugaresi E, eds. *Migraine and epilepsy*. Boston: Butterworths; 1987:189–201.
7. Gibbs EL, Gibbs FA. Extreme spindles: correlation of electroencephalographic sleep pattern with mental retardation. *Science* 1962;138:1106–1107.

Alternating Hemiplegia of Childhood, edited by
Frederick Andermann, Jean Aicardi, and Federico Vigevano,
Raven Press, Ltd., New York © 1995.

13

Single Photon Emission Computed Tomography Studies in Alternating Hemiplegia of Childhood

Mary L. Zupanc*, Scott B. Perlman†, and Robert S. Rust†

*Department of Neurology, Division of Child Neurology, Mayo Clinic,
200 SW First Avenue, Rochester, MN 55905; and †Department of Radiology and
Neurology, University of Wisconsin Hospital and Clinics, 600 Highland Avenue,
Madison, WI 53792.*

SPECT IMAGING IN CHILDREN USING CEREBRAL PERFUSION RADIOTRACERS

Single photon emission computed tomography (SPECT) of brain with intravenous radiotracers has proven an accurate method for evaluation of cerebral perfusion. Appropriate radiotracers and SPECT equipment are available in the imaging departments of most tertiary medical centers. The technique has been used to obtain clinically useful information in many neurologic disorders of adults including epilepsy, dementia, and cerebrovascular disease. The most common application of this procedure in children has been for the evaluation of cerebral perfusion in patients with medically intractable seizures.

The two most commonly used radiotracers for evaluation of regional cerebral perfusion are ^{123}I-labeled N-isopropyl-4-iodo-amphetamine (IMP), and technetium-99m-labeled ([99]mTc-) hexamethylpropylene amine oxime (HMPAO). IMP is a lipophilic agent with high brain penetration after intravenous injection. Regional uptake and retention are proportional to regional cerebral perfusion. Possible mechanisms responsible for brain retention of these radiotracers include protein binding or conversion to a more polar form under the influence of intracellular pH as the result of enzymatic processes, particularly changes of the isopropyl side chain (1). Brain saturation is also maintained by redistribution of unmetabolized IMP from lungs and fat to brain, counterbalancing the slow clearance of brain amphetamine (2). Thus, the net result of these effects is that the overall amount of brain radiotracer concentration remains constant and proportional to initial cerebral perfusion for up to 60 minutes after bolus injection, the interval during which SPECT images of brain are acquired.

HMPAO, a ^{99m}Tc radiopharmaceutical, is also lipid-soluble and readily crosses intact blood-brain barrier. HMPAO reaction with intracellular glutathione quickly traps the radiotracer within the brain (1). As with IMP, the cerebral uptake is proportional to regional cerebral blood flow. A significant advantage of this radiotracer over IMP is that HMPAO is retained much longer by the brain, showing no significant washout from the brain for up to 8 hours after bolus intravenous administration (2). Thus, images reflecting central blood flow at the time of HMPAO administration can be obtained several hours later. Another major advantage of HMPAO is the availability of kits that permit HMPAO labelling with ^{99m}Tc as needed. Prelabeled IMP must be ordered in advance and deteriorates with prolonged storage.

SPECT sensitivity in detection of regional differences in blood flow with either tracer has greatly improved with the availability of multidetector SPECT arrays.

SPECT brain perfusion examinations play an important role in children in the localization of epileptogenic foci (3–8). Useful information has been obtained with both interictal and ictal SPECT (9,10).

In one series of 56 children with epilepsy, interictal HMPAO SPECT of brain provided important information in 79%. Among 22 children with partial epilepsy arising from a well defined focus, SPECT demonstrated hypoperfusion in 21 and increased perfusion in just one. This patient had continuous epileptiform activity at the time of investigation (3).

SPECT imaging of cerebral perfusion in children has also been applied to the study of other diseases, including stroke (3), encephalopathy (3), and alternating hemiplegia of childhood (AHC) (11).

SPECT IMAGING IN CHILDREN WITH ALTERNATING HEMIPLEGIA OF CHILDHOOD

The pathophysiology of AHC with its paroxysmal episodes of tonic or atonic hemiplegia is not clearly understood. Some authors have hypothesized that AHC is related to migraine because of its paroxysmal nature and its clinical similarity to hemiplegic (complicated) migraine (12). Others have suggested that it represents an atypical, intractable form of epilepsy (12–14). SPECT brain imaging has been performed on several children with AHC during, immediately after, or remote from acute hemiplegic attacks. SPECT, as a well standardized method for evaluation of regional cerebral blood flow, has particular advantages in evaluation of AHC. Thus, if AHC is migrainous or involves spreading cortical depression, this technique should disclose diminished cerebral perfusion of the involved hemisphere during a hemiplegic episode. On the other hand, if AHC represents a form of epilepsy, ictal SPECT should demonstrate increased cerebral perfusion of the involved hemisphere due to the increased metabolic rate and glucose demands, provoking increased blood flow. The results of SPECT brain imaging in two patients with alternating hemiplegia are described below.

CASE REPORT 1

MP was the full-term product of a normal pregnancy, labor and delivery. Her perinatal history was unremarkable. She first sat at age 10 months and walked with support at 20 months. She is now 7 years old and shows significant cognitive and motor delay. She has approximately 70 words in her vocabulary. She can play only simple games such as peek-a-boo. She requires assistance in all daily living skills, e.g., eating and dressing. She is able to walk, except during acute episodes of hemiplegia. Her gait is, however, unsteady and wide-based.

Her hemiplegic episodes started at about five months of age. Characteristically, they begin with tonic stiffening of either the right or the left side, often accompanied by tonic eye deviation to the ipsilateral side. Occasionally, oculogyric movements are seen. The tonic phase lasts for minutes to hours, and is invariably followed by flaccid ipsilateral hemiparesis which lasts for hours to days. Mild choreiform movements may appear concomitantly. Episodes are often accompanied by dysphagia. Episodes of right hemiplegia are always accompanied by expressive aphasia. The episodes initially occurred weekly but subsequently increased in frequency to almost daily.

Between the episodes, MP's neurological examination is significant for poor cognitive function for age; intact cranial nerve function; diffuse spasticity and hyperreflexia, emphasized in the lower extremities; and wide-based gait.

Laboratory studies, including fluorescent antibody panel (antinuclear antibody, antimitochondrial antibody, and antiparietal antibody), sedimentation rate, serum lactate and pyruvate, plasma and urine amino acids, urine organic acids, blood lead level, routine serum chemistry, and CBC with differential were all normal. CSF cell count, glucose, and protein were normal. Brain CT and MRI scans with contrast, as well as cerebral angiography were normal. Numerous interictal EEGs were normal. Ictal EEGs have invariably shown slowing of the hemisphere contralateral to the acute hemiparesis. Electron microscopy of a skin biopsy showed no abnormalities. Muscle biopsy was normal with no evidence of mitochondrial abnormalities on electron microscopy. Qualitative staining of muscle for electron chain enzymes was normal. Quantitative assays of the muscle for electron chain enzymes were also normal.

Standard anticonvulsant medications (phenobarbital, valproic acid, carbamazepine), verapamil, Benadryl, and Cogentin did not result in any change in the frequency, severity or duration of the spells. Flunarizine (15 mg/d) has resulted in a marked reduction in the severity, frequency, and duration of her hemiplegic episodes. At present she is having only one severe episode of hemiplegia per month with milder episodes at weekly intervals.

METHODS AND RESULTS

SPECT using ^{123}I-iodoamphetamine was performed to further evaluate her brain perfusion. She was studied twice, once during an acute episode of right hemiplegia

(5–6 hours after onset) and again when she had recovered from that episode, several days later.

These studies were performed with a GE Star II SPECT gamma camera equipped with a 30 degree slant-hole collimator. Three mCi of ^{123}I-IMP (Medi-Physics, Inc.), produced initially by the (p, 2n) and later the (p, 5n) reaction, was injected into an arm vein while she was lying in a dark, quiet room. She was subsequently sedated with 60 mg/kg of oral chloral hydrate. Her eyes remained closed throughout the procedure. Data acquisition started 20 minutes after injection. Sixty-four projections at 40 seconds per projection were used for data acquisition, yielding an average imaging time of about 40 minutes. Images were acquired into a 128×128 matrix. Reconstruction was performed with a Butterworth filter at a cutoff frequency of 0.41 and a power of 10. Linear attenuation correction was performed with a calculated value of $0.12 \ \text{cm}^{-1}$. Images were then analyzed qualitatively for differential regional iodoamphetamine uptake.

SPECT brain images obtained during the right hemiplegic episode (Fig. 1) showed hypoperfusion of the entire left cerebral hemisphere. Re-examination after resolution of her hemiplegia (Fig. 1) showed normal, unilaterally symmetrical brain perfusion (15).

CASE REPORT 2

TD was the full term product of a normal pregnancy. There were no perinatal problems except for:

1. A possible "seizure" consisting of transient back extension and stiffening of the extremities. Her neonatal EEG was normal.
2. Intermittent primary gaze nystagmus with a normal ophthalmologic exam, and
3. Mild generalized hypotonia.

Initial developmental milestones were normal. By 20 months old she was sitting independently but not standing or walking. She did not speak, but clearly understood a few words. She was hypotonic, but her neurological examination was otherwise unremarkable except during episodes of acute hemiplegia.

At 4 months of age, TD had a second episode of extremity stiffening, lasting 20–30 seconds and accompanied by "staring." This occurred 24 hours after a DPT booster. An EEG was normal.

At 7 months of age, she developed neck weakness losing the ability to hold up her head. She also developed bilateral upper extremity flaccidity, lethargy, and irritability, all of which persisted for 1 week. Subsequently, she has had frequent, briefer hemiplegic episodes, occurring every 2 days and lasting 20–30 minutes. TD's episodes are sometimes precipitated by stress or fatigue. They began with irritability followed by loss of neck strength and marked weakness of either the right or the left side of the body (arm much greater than leg). Some episodes became unilateral. When tested, hemianopsia ipsilateral to the weakness was clearly pres-

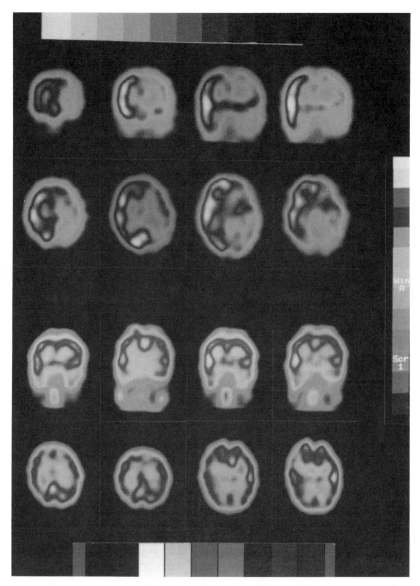

FIG. 1. (Upper 2 rows) Static SPECT images of case 1 during an episode of right hemiplegia study was performed with a GE Star II SPECT gamma camera equipped with a 30° slant hole collinator. Images were obtained 20 minutes following intravenous injection of 3mCi of [128]I-IMP. These images demonstrate hypoperfusion of the entire left cerebral hemisphere. **(Lower 2 rows)** Repeat static SPECT image of this patient when she was at baseline. The study demonstrates no perfusion abnormalities. (From Zupanc et al., ref. 11, with permission.)

ent. Weakness was followed by increased irritability, crying, and brief transient dystonia. Occasionally, flurries of primary gaze nystagmus were noted during episodes. The hemiplegia resolved after 20–30 minutes.

Laboratory studies (as in Case 1) were all normal. MRI scans of the brain and cervical spine were normal. MRI angiography of the brain and cervical spine was normal. Interictal EEGs have all been normal. Ictal EEGs have either been normal or have shown mild slowing of the hemisphere contralateral to acute hemiparesis.

TD has never received anticonvulsant medication. She is currently receiving flunarizine 5 mg/d. In the initial 3 months, the hemiplegic episodes have been reduced from daily events to once or twice every 2 to 3 weeks.

METHODS AND RESULTS

SPECT brain imaging was performed during and after resolution of an acute hemiplegic episode. Injection was performed less than 20 minutes after onset of hemiparesis. The same methodology was applied as in case report 1, except that a different isotope, HMPAO—was used to determine cerebral perfusion.

SPECT brain images obtained during the right hemiplegic episode demonstrated near absence of perfusion over the entire left cerebral hemisphere as well as the left cerebellar hemisphere (Fig. 2). After resolution of the hemiparesis, the asymmetry in cerebral perfusion resolved completely.

DISCUSSION

In these two patients, we observed transient, reversible hypoperfusion of the cerebral hemisphere contralateral to the hemiplegia. In one patient these changes were measured in closer proximity to the onset of a hemiplegic episode than in any other patient heretofore reported. These findings show diminished blood flow, and if taken together with the ictal EEG findings, suggest hypometabolism.

These changes do not correspond with those usually observed in acute focal epilepsy, where SPECT shows increased blood flow and the EEG shows electrographic seizures.

Our results are consistent with those obtained by Aicardi and colleagues. Studies of two patients showed cerebral hypoperfusion of the hemisphere contralateral to hemiparesis during an acute episode (Aicardi, *personal communication*, 1992). Nevšímalová and colleagues have have performed SPECT brain imaging using ^{99m}Tc-HMPAO in six patients with AHC, but only one of these was an ictal study. This patient also had cerebral hypoperfusion contralateral to hemiparesis (Nevšímalová, *personal communication*, 1992). Rho and colleagues have reported fluctuating bihemispheric and contralateral hemispheric blood flow in a single patient with AHC, improving on flunarizine therapy (16).

Strashun, Aminian, and Rose have recently reported six ^{99m}Tc-HMPAO SPECT imaging studies of three patients that showed *hyperperfusion* of the contralateral cerebral hemisphere late in the course of hemiplegic attacks, typically several hours

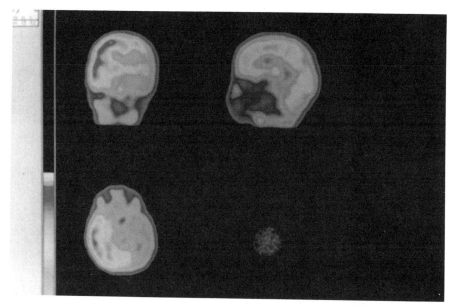

FIG. 2. Static SPECT images of case report 2 during an episode of right hemiplegia. The same methodology was applied as in case report 1, except that a different isotope was used to determine cerebral perfusion, i.e., HMPAO-hexamethylpropylenamine oxime. These images demonstrate near absence of perfusion over the entire left cerebral hemisphere.

after the onset of hemiplegia (17). Two interictal SPECT studies showed normal and symmetric cerebral perfusion. It is possible that the very different but consistent images represent a phase of cerebral perfusion late in attacks, possibly representing a form of "luxury perfusion" after relative insufficiency of cerebral blood flow, as seen in our patients. Support for such a view is provided by ictal ^{1}H-MR spectroscopy showing evidence for energy failure during the early acute phase of AHC and normal interictal spectroscopy (18).

Kanazawa and colleagues reported two ictal ^{99m}TC-HMPAO SPECT studies in a patient with presumed AHC (19). Both ictal scans showed cerebral hyperperfusion contralateral to the acute hemiplegia. However, the case report of this young 12-month-old boy is quite unusual and atypical for children with AHC. Recurrent episodes of right or left *hand* palsy are described rather than typical episodes of hemiplegia. One of these SPECT brain imaging studies was performed more than 24 hours after the onset of the hand palsy.

CONCLUSION

The use of SPECT brain imaging in patients with alternating hemiplegia has provided important pathophysiologic information. The finding of hypoperfusion of the involved hemisphere early in the course of an episode suggests one of several possible conclusions. First, primary failure of blood supply because of vascular dysfunction but secondary cerebral energy failure may occur. Second, diminuation of hemispheric circulation may merely represent blood flow reduction after depression (e.g., spreading cortical depression) of cortical metabolic activity. In the first, uncoupling of blood flow and metabolism occurs. In the second, these remain coupled, but cerebral events are responsible for the transient neurologic dysfunction. A primary disturbance of cerebral energy metabolism is supported by our metabolic (^{1}H-MR spectroscopy) studies (18). Treatment with flunarizine, a calcium channel blocker which has been shown to both protect brain cells from hypoxic-ischemic injury and to prevent vasospasm, has resulted in marked improvement in our children with alternating hemiplegia. Thus, this drug may be protective whether vascular or metabolic defects are primary in AHC. Clearly, our results do not support the argument that AHC is an epileptic condition. Rather, they support that AHC may be more closely related to changes in cerebral blood flow and/or metabolism, as has been suggested by others (20–22).

REFERENCES

1. Kung HF, Ohmomo Y, Kung M. Current and future radiopharmaceuticals for brain imaging with single photon emission computed tomography. *Sem Nucl Med* 1990;xx:290–302.
2. Holman BL, Moretti J, Hill T. Brain imaging with radiolabeled amines and other perfusion tracers. In: Gottschalk A, Hoffer PB, Potchen EJ, eds. *Diagnostic Nuclear Medicine.* Baltimore: Williams and Wilkins; 1988:899–913.
3. Uvebrant P, Bjure J, Hedstrom A, Ekholm S. Brain single photon emission computed tomography (SPECT) in neuropediatrics. *Neuropediatrics* 1991;22:3–9.
4. Adams C, Hwang PA, Gilday DL, et al. Comparison of SPECT, EEG, CT, MRI, and pathology in partial epilepsy. *Pediatr Neurol* 1992;8:97–103.
5. Chiron C, Raynaud C, Dulac O, et al. Study of the cerebral blood flow in partial epilepsy of childhood using the SPECT method. *J Neuroradiol* 1989;16:317–324.
6. Hara M, Takahashi M, Kojima A, et al. Single photon emission computed tomography in children with idiopathic seizures. *Radiat Med* 1991;9:185–189.
7. Abdel-Dayem HM, Nawaz MK, Hassoon MM, et al. Cerebral perfusion abnormalities in therapy-resistant epilepsy in mentally retarded pediatric patients. Comparison between EEG, X-ray CT, and Tc-99m HMPAO. *Clin Nucl Med* 1991;16:557–561.
8. Konkol RJ, Maister BH, Wells RG, Sty JR. Hemimegalencephaly: Clinical, EEG, neuroimaging, and IMP-SPECT correlation. *Pediatr Neurol* 1990;6;414–418.
9. Rowe CC, Berkovic SF, Austin M, McKay WJ, Bladin PF. Postictal scan in epilepsy [Letter]. *Lancet* 1989;1(8634):389–390.
10. Lee BI, Markand ON, Wellman HN, et al. HIPDM-SPECT in patients with medically intractable complex partial seizures. *Arch Neurol* 1988;45:397–402.
11. Zupanc ML, Dobkin JA, Perlman SB. I-123–iodoamphetamine SPECT brain imaging in alternating hemiplegia. *Pediatr Neurol* 1991;7:35–38.
12. Aicardi J, Krägeloh I. Alternating hemiplegia in infants. Report of five cases. *Dev Med Child Neurol* 1980;22:784–790.
13. Verret S, Steele JC. Alternating hemiplegia in childhood. *Pediatrics* 1971;47(4):675–679.
14. Hosking GP, Cavanagh NPC, Wilson J. Alternating hemiplegia: complicated migraine of infancy. *Arch Dis Child* 1978;53:656–659.
15. Dittrich J, Havlóva M, Nevšímalová S. Paroxysmal hemiparesis in childhood. *Dev Med Child Neurol* 1979;21:800–806.
16. Rho JM, Mena I, Migneco O, et al. Improvement in regional cerebral blood flow after Flunarizine therapy in a patient with alternating hemiplegia. *Ann Neurol* 1992;32(3):451–452.

17. Strashun A, Aminian A, Rose A. SPECT imaging in alternating hemiplegia. *Nuclear Medicine* 1992;33:1021–1022.
18. Rust RS, Thomas A, Zupanc ML, et al. ^{1}H Volume localized in vivo MR spectroscopy and SPECT alternating hemiplegia (AH). *Ann Neurol* 1992;32(3):452.
19. Kanazawa, Shirasaka Y, Hattori H, Okuno I, Mikawa H. Ictal ^{99m}TC-HMPAO SPECT in alternating hemiplegia. *Pediatr Neurol* 1991;7:121–124.
20. Casaer P. Flunarizine in alternating hemiplegia in childhood. An international study in twelve children. *Neuropediatrics* 1987;18(4):191–195.
21. Holmes B, Brodgen RN, Heel RC, Speight TM, Avery GS. Flunarizine: a review of its pharmacodynamic and pharmacokinetic properties and therapeutic use. *Drugs* 1984;27:6–44.
22. Casaer P. Flunarizine in alternating hemiplegia in childhood. *Lancet* 1984;2:579.

Alternating Hemiplegia of Childhood, edited by
Frederick Andermann, Jean Aicardi, and Federico Vigevano,
Raven Press, Ltd., New York © 1995.

14

Positron Emission Tomography in Children with Alternating Hemiplegia of Childhood

Mohamad A. Mikati* and Alan J. Fischman**

*Department of Neurology, *Children's Hospital, Harvard Medical School, 300 Longwood Avenue, Boston, MA 02115; and Department of Radiology, **Harvard Medical School, Massachusetts General Hospital, 32 Fruit Street, Boston, MA 02114.*

Positron emission tomography (PET) is based on the principle of detecting photons emitted after the annihilation of an emitted positron with an electron (1). A number of positron emitting radiopharmaceuticals can be given to patients to obtain images which reflect specific physiologic precesses. The most commonly used agent is 2-deoxy-2[^{18}F]fluoro-D-glucose (FDG) which is used to estimate the cerebral metabolic rate. The brain utilizes glucose as its primary source of energy. Hence a map of brain glucose utilization is considered to reflect the rate of cerebral metabolism. FDG is transported through the blood-brain barrier like glucose. It is also similarly metabolized by the enzyme hexokinase and is consequently trapped intracellularly in the brain. It is however not metabolized through the glycolytic pathway and thus does not interfere with normal cerebral metabolism. Emissions from labeled FDG can be used to calculate, based on specific models, numerical estimates of the cerebral glucose metabolic rate (CMRGlc). More frequently in clinical situations maps of relative CMRGlc are obtained. The comparison of relative emissions of ^{18}F from different areas of the brain allows for comparison of relative CMRGlc in those areas.

PET scanning can also be utilized to determine cerebral blood flow and cerebral rate of oxygen metabolism (CMRO$_2$) (1). This requires the use of the isotope ^{15}O. Intravenous H$_2$^{15}O allows the performance of those measurements. Administration of C^{15}O$_2$ by inhalation, which is converted in the lung to H$_2$^{15}O by carbonic anhydrase, allows the measurement of cerebral blood flow. Related PET techniques can also be used to measure cerebral blood volume and oxygen extraction fraction.

PET investigations of different central nervous system disorders have revealed distinctive abnormalities in different entities. This has allowed better understanding of the pathophysiology of those disorders and in many cases helped in the differential diagnosis and in the clinical management of patients.

Several types of dementing encephalopathies have been investigated with PET

(1). Patients with multi-infarct dementia have multiple areas of hypometabolism. Patients with Alzheimer's disease usually have a typical pattern of parietal, temporal, and frontal hypometabolism with sparing of other cerebral areas and of deep structures. Patients with depression and "pseudodementia" usually have normal PET scans (1). In childhood encephalopathies PET imaging has also been useful. For example, children with Lennox-Gastaut syndrome have a diffuse decrease in CMRGlc while those with partial epilepsy have focal abnormalities (2). Children with a number of inborn errors of metabolism (dihydropteridine reductase deficiency, phenylketonuria, and cytochrome c oxidase deficiency) have reduced CMRGlc in the caudate and putamen (2).

Epileptic foci typically have decreased metabolism interictally and increased metabolism with increased blood flow ictally (3–5). Postictally an extension of the area of hypometabolism to contiguous areas has been reported. PET scans are more sensitive in detecting epileptic foci than CT scans. The metabolic abnormality is usually more extensive than the anatomic lesion detected preoperatively by MRI imaging, or postoperatively by pathologic examination of the resected tissue. In one study 15/17 patients with unilateral electroencephalographic epileptic foci had focal or lateralized areas of hypometabolism (4). Focal PET scan abnormalities, detected quantitatively, can be a useful prognostic indicator prior to surgical resection of temporal lobe foci (5). Generalized epilepsies on the other hand have been reported to show normal PET scans interictally and generalized abnormalities (hypo or hypermetabolism) ictally (6).

During hemiplegia resulting from strokes a specific sequence of abnormalities has been described. There is initially an increase in cerebral blood volume, despite a decrease in cerebral blood flow, due to compensatory vasodilation. Further decrease in cerebral blood flow is followed by an increase in the oxygen extraction fraction while the $CMRO_2$ remains constant. With further compromise in cerebral blood flow there is a decrease in $CMRO_2$ and an infarct results. During the infarct the cerebral blood flow may occasionally increase (hyperemic infarct), and the oxygen extraction fraction may also be variable (1). Subsequent luxury perfusion almost always occurs (7). These focal PET abnormalities occur in regions that correspond to the expected functional anatomic localization in the hemisphere contralateral to the neurological deficit (8,9). However widespread metabolic depression is formed in areas remote from the territory of the obstructed vessel (e.g., middle cerebral artery), including other cortical areas, the thalamus ipsilaterally, and the cerebellar hemisphere contralaterally. Additionally patients with lacunar infarcts usually do not show PET abnormalities (8). PET investigations have shown that after hemiplegia resulting from a contralateral stroke ipsilateral motor pathways play an important role in the recovery of function of the hemiplegic limb (10).

There has been only limited experience with PET studies in patients with migraine (11–13). Cerebral blood flow changes with no variations in $CMRO_2$ have been reported in patients with neurologic manifestations during migraine attacks. Parenteral administration of reserpine to precipitate migraine headaches has been associated with a bilateral and diffuse reduction of CMRGlc even before the headache starts (11).

We have performed FDG PET studies on three patients with sporadic (non-familial) AHC. All patients had clinical features consistent with those typical of the syndrome as described by Aicardi (14). All three also had negative extensive metabolic workups, MRIs, and MRI angiography studies. The first patient was a 15-month-old boy whose initial symptoms started at age one day when he developed recurrent episodes of abnormal eye movements. When seen at the age of 18 months he was having weekly episodes of unilateral or bilateral hemiplegia since the age of 9 months. Associated nystagmoid eye movements were noted during the spells. Each hemiplegic episode lasted several days and manifested fluctuations with transient remissions of a few minutes duration occurring mainly after awakening from sleep. Developmentally he was at approximately the 11-month level. The patient was investigated in the asymptomatic state and before he was started on flunarizine therapy. Approximately 45 minutes after the administration of 142 MBq [18]-FDG, tomographic images of the brain were obtained and did not reveal any abnormalities. The second patient was a 44-month-old girl whose abnormal eye movements started at the age of 2 months and lasted till the age of 26 months. Episodes of alternating hemiplegia started at approximately the age of two years and occurred once every 2 to 3 months. She too was investigated while not receiving medications. Developmentally she was at approximately the 2-½ year level. Approximately 45 minutes after the administration of 115 MBq [18]-FDG, tomographic images of the brain were obtained. These revealed normal cerebral metabolism with no asymmetry (Fig. 1). The third patient was the most severely affected. She was a 49-month-old girl whose episodes of tonic stiffening started in the neonatal period and continued thereafter. At the age of one year the episodes of hemiplegia started. When examined at the age of 49 months she had severe developmental delay with a functional level of approximately 14 months. She still could not walk. Her neurological examination revealed bilateral hyperreflexia with bilateral extensor plantar responses. Her episodes of alternating hemiplegia were occurring weekly, each usually lasting several days at a time. During one of her attacks she had been admitted to a local hospital and had suffered a respiratory arrest after receiving large doses of benzodiazepines. A PET scan was carried out several months later while she was receiving flunarizine, clonazepam, and acetazolamide. Approximately 45 minutes after the administration of 144 MBq [18]-FDG, tomographic images of the brain were obtained. The scan revealed symmetrical and apparently normal cerebral metabolism, but there was a decrease in the metabolic activity of the cerebellum, diffusely, relative to the cerebrum (Fig. 2). This latter finding was of uncertain significance. Her MRI at that time was normal.

Tada et al. reported an 11-year-old boy with AHC who was studied with PET using $C^{15}O_2$. The scan revealed a slight decrease of cerebral blood flow in the insula, putamen, and claustrum of the left side during a right-sided hemiplegic episode (15). Measurement of regional cerebral blood flow by ^{133}Xe inhalation method revealed a slight bilateral decrease in cerebral blood flow during a quadriplegic episode.

These findings tend to favor a vascular rather than an epileptic etiology for the hemiplegic spells. Interictal hypometabolic focal changes, characteristic of focal

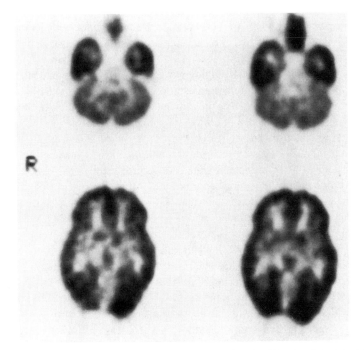

FIG. 1. PET scan of a 32-month-old girl with AHC in the interictal (nonhemiplegic) state. Cuts shown are at the level of the cerebellum and temporal lobe and at the level of the thalamus and lower basal ganglia. No significant asymmetries or focal findings are noted.

epilepsy were not seen in the three AHC patients. In addition, the one available ictal study revealed hypo rather than hyperperfusion during an attack. On the other hand Casaer reported ictal and interictal PET abnormalities in the frontal lobe and in the thalamus (16). The latter findings underscore the need for more studies in this syndrome particularly with ictal scans at various stages of the hemiplegia, dystonia, seizures, and posturing spells. Such studies should make it possible to better understand the pathophysiology underlying the various types of movement abnormalities noted in AHC. In addition, interictal studies could complement the ictal investigations and perhaps help better characterize the encephalopathy that accompanies this syndrome.

SUMMARY

This chapter reported the results of PET studies performed by us and reviewed those performed by other investigators on patients with AHC. The utility of this technique in evaluating other disorders related to AHC, and in providing potential insights into the pathophysiology of those disorders and of AHC was also reviewed. Only a few PET investigations have been performed on patients with AHC. In our

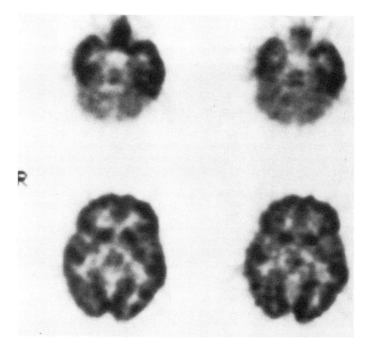

FIG. 2. PET scan of a 38-month-old girl with AHC in the interictal (nonhemiplegic) state. Cuts shown are at the level of the cerebellum and temporal lobe and at the level of the lower basal ganglia. There is an apparent relative decrease in the cerebellar metabolic rate. There is a mild tilt apparent on the temporal lobe level cuts.

experience interictal 2-deoxy-2[^{18}F]fluoro-D-glucose (FDG) studies have revealed symmetrical cerebral metabolism. Evidence for bilateral cerebellar hypometabolism in one patient was noted. Hypometabolic changes similar to those seen interictally in patients with epileptic foci were not present. An ictal ^{15}O scan performed by another group revealed hypoperfusion of the basal ganglia contralateral to the hemiplegia. These findings favor a vascular rather than an epileptic etiology of the attacks. PET studies of patients with AHC may help improve our understanding of the pathophysiology of that disorder, but more investigations are needed.

ACKNOWLEDGMENT

Supported in part by the Wark epilepsy research fund (MAM).

REFERENCES

1. Hawkins RA, Phelps ME. Positron emission tomography for evaluation of cerebral function. *Current Concepts in Diagnostic Nuclear Medicine* 1986;3:4–13.
2. Yanai K, Iinuma K, Matsuzawa T, Ito M, Miyabayashi S, Narisawa K, Ido T, Yamada K, Tada K.

Cerebral glucose utilization in pediatric neurological disorders determined by positron emission tomography. *Eur J Nucl Med* 1987;13:292–296.
3. Engel J Jr., Brown WJ, Kuhl DE, et al. Pathological findings underlying focal temporal lobe hypometabolism in partial epilepsy. *Ann Neurol* 1982;12:518–528.
4. Theodore WH, Brooks R, Sato S, Patronas N, Margolin R, DiChiro G, Porter RJ. The role of positron emission tomography in the evaluation of seizure disorders. *Ann Neurol* 1984;15(Suppl): S176–179.
5. Theodore WH, Sato S, Kufta C, Balish MB, Bromfield EB, Leiderman DB. Temporal lobectomy for uncontrolled seizures: the role of positron emission tomography. *Ann Neurol* 1992;32:789–794.
6. Theodore WH, Brooks R, Margolin R, Patronas N, Sato S, Porter RJ, Mansi L, Bairamian D, DiChiro G. Positron emission tomography in generalized seizures. *Neurology* 1985;35:684–690.
7. Baron JC, Bousser MG, Comar D, Rougemont D, Lebrun-Grandie P, Castaigne P. Positron emission tomography in the physiopathological study of cerebral ischemia in man. *Presse Med* 1983; 12:3066–3072.
8. Rougemont D, Baron JC, Lebrun-Grandie P, Bousser MG, Soisson T, Comar D. A¹5 oxygen positron study of relative local perfusion and oxygen extraction of the brain in lacunar hemiparesis. *Pathol Biol (Paris)* 1982;30:295–302.
9. Heiss WD, Vyska K, Kloster G, Traupe H, Freundlieb C, Hoeck A, Feinendegen LE, Stoecklin G. Demonstration of decreased functional activity of visual cortex by [¹¹C]methylglucose and positron emission tomography. *Neuroradiology* 1982;23:45–47.
10. Chollet F, DiPiero V, Wise RJ, Brooks DJ, Dolan RJ, Frackowiak RS. The functional anatomy of motor recovery after stroke in humans: a study with positron emission tomography. *Ann Neurol* 1991;29:63–71.
11. Sachs H, Russell JA, Christman DR, Fowler JS, Wolf AP. Positron emission tomographic studies on induced migraine [Letter]. *Lancet* 1984;2(8400):465.
12. Bousser MG, Baron JC. Importance of positron emission tomography for the study of cerebral ischemia. *Ann Med Interne (Paris)* 1981;132:449–455.
13. Chabriat H. Positron emission tomography and migraine. *Pathol Biol (Paris)* 1992;40:344–348.
14. Bourgeois M, Aicardi J, Goutières F. Alternating hemiplegia of childhood. *J Pediatr* 1993;122: 673–679.
15. Tada H, Miyake S, Yamada M, Iwamoto H, Morooka K, Sakuragawa N. A patient with alternating hemiplegia in childhood. *No To Hattatsu* 1989;21:283–288.
16. Casaer P. PET scanning in alternating hemiplegia of childhood. *Presented at the International Workshop on Alternating Hemiplegia of Childhood*. Rome, January 1992.

Alternating Hemiplegia of Childhood, edited by
Frederick Andermann, Jean Aicardi, and Federico Vigevano,
Raven Press, Ltd., New York © 1995.

15

Mitochondrial Dysfunction in Patients with Alternating Hemiplegia of Childhood

Fluctuation Over Time in Relation to Clinical State

Nicola De Stefano, *Kenneth Silver, Frederick Andermann, and
Douglas L. Arnold

*Departments of Neurology, Neurosurgery, and Pediatrics, McGill University, Montreal,
Quebec H3A 2B4, Canada; and *Montreal Children's Hospital, Montreal Neurological
Hospital and Institute, 3801 University Street, Montreal, Quebec H3H 1P3, Canada.*

Magnetic resonance (MR) spectroscopy (MRS) is a sensitive and noninvasive method for studying metabolism *in vivo* (1–3). Phosphorus spectra contain resonances from most of the important phosphate-containing intermediates of cellular energy metabolism. The phosphorus MR spectrum of normal muscle (Fig. 1) consists of five major peaks: three from adenosine triphosphate (ATP), one from phosphocreatine (PCr) and one from inorganic phosphate (P_i). The intracellular pH can be determined from the position of the P_i peak. Knowledge of these metabolite concentrations allows calculation of metabolically active cytosolic adenosine diphosphate (ADP) as well as the cytosolic phosphorylation potential (PP), an important index of the amount of energy mitochondria are able to store in ATP. Since the main function of mitochondria is to provide chemical energy for metabolism by means of synthesis of ATP from ADP and P_i and maintain a high PP, phosphorus MRS provides a unique tool to study mitochondrial function *in vivo* and to detect mitochondrial dysfunction. Proton MR spectra obtained at relatively long echo time (TE 272) reveal four major resonances: one originating mainly from choline-containing phospholipids (Cho) involved in membrane metabolism, one from creatine (Cr) either free or in phosphocreatine, one from *N*-acetylaspartate (NAA), a neuronal marker (4,5), and one from lactate (LA), the product of anaerobic glycolysis and an indirect index of oxidative metabolism.

We recently reported evidence of mitochondrial dysfunction in patients with al-

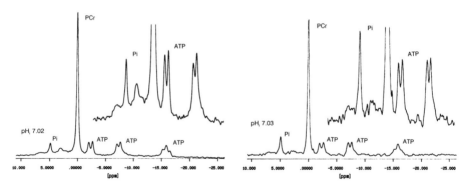

FIG. 1. Phosphorus MR spectrum of resting calf muscle in a normal subject (left) and in a patient with AHC (right).

ternating hemiplegia of childhood (AHC) and suggested that this represents a previously unrecognized phenotype of mitochondrial cytopathy (6). In this chapter we provide further evidence of mitochondrial dysfunction in muscle in three of the four originally described patients with AHC and describe fluctuations over time corresponding to clinical and treatment status over 3 years. In addition, we describe abnormalities in proton MRS of brain consistent with neuronal damage and loss.

MATERIALS AND METHODS

Patients

Three patients were examined over a 3-year follow-up period. During this time phosphorus MRS examination of muscle was performed on three occasions in two subjects and on two occasions in one (patient 2). Proton spectroscopy of brain was performed in patient 2 on two occasions 1 year apart.

All patients fulfilled the diagnostic criteria of Aicardi (7), i.e., all had onset before the age of 18 months, recurrent attacks of hemiplegia involving either or both sides, paroxysmal dystonic attacks, and cognitive impairment.

The three patients formed part of the group of four whose initial MRS findings we described previously. One of these four patients, who remained cognitively unimpaired, has a sibling who now also has developed AHC. This patient has now been diagnosed as having benign familial nocturnal AHC and is described separately in this volume (see Chapter 17). MRS was also performed in a patient with alternating paroxysmal dystonia and hemiplegia symptomatic of basal ganglia disease presented in this volume (see Chapter 19) and in a child with alternating hemiplegia as a manifestation of pyruvate dehydrogenase deficiency reported by Silver et al. (see Chapter 20).

MRS

Muscle

Phosphorus MR spectra were obtained from resting gastrocnemius muscle using a 1.5 Tesla combined imaging and spectroscopy system (Philips, Best, The Netherlands) and a 6 cm surface coil. The time between pulses (TR) was 30 seconds. Under these conditions, resonance or peak intensity in the MR spectrum is directly proportional to metabolite concentration *in vivo*. Resonance intensities were determined using a model-based, nonlinear optimization routine operating in the time domain (8).

Concentrations of P_i and PCr were calculated from resonance intensities relative to the mean resonance intensity for the three resonances of ATP, not including the overlapping resonance from nicotine adenine dinucleotide which was fitted separately. ATP was assumed to have a concentration of 8 mM in intracellular water (9,10). Intracellular pH was determined from the chemical shift of P_i, using a previously determined titration curve (11). The concentration of free, metabolically active ADP in the cytoplasm was determined from the creatine kinase equilibrium, as previously described (12). The phosphorylation potential was calculated from the ratio $[ATP]/[ADP][P_i]$.

Brain

Proton spectra of brain were obtained using a 90°-180°-180° sequence to select a large central periventricular volume of interest (VOI) with dimensions 90 mm $AP \times 74$ mm $LR \times 24$ mm CC. The water signal was suppressed by selective inversion of the water prior to acquiring the spectrum as the water signal passed through zero. Two hundred fifty-six transients were averaged with an interpulse delay of 2 seconds and an echo time of 272 milliseconds.

Statistics

The Kruskall-Wallis test of variance was employed for the analysis of data from muscle. For both muscle and brain, data were considered significant if the probability of difference was less than 0.05.

RESULTS

Muscle MR results for the three patients with AHC were compared with those for 34 normal adult control subjects. MR spectra of muscle from children older than about one year are similar to those of adults (L. Bertocci, *personal communication*,

1992). The first examination of the patients' muscle had a mean concentration of P_i and ADP that was abnormally high and a mean PCr concentration and PP that was abnormally low with respect to normal subjects (Table 1). Metabolite values fluctuated over time to a greater extent in the patients than in normal subjects ($p < 0.001$) and appeared to improve or deteriorate in relation to clinical and treatment status as described below.

Brain MR results for patient 2 were compared with those of 18 normal adult control subjects in whom the same VOI was selected.

Patient 1

This 6-year-old girl was born after a normal pregnancy and delivery. At 3 months of age she developed episodes of head and eye turning to the left with unilateral nystagmus and irritable screaming. Hemiplegic attacks started at 9 months of age and involved one arm or leg or both sides with coldness and pallor of the extremities and dystonic posturing of the foot. Attacks lasted for several hours, but if she slept for a few minutes the hemiparesis would be resolved on awakening.

She was initially assessed at 4 years of age. Flunarizine 5 mg twice daily resulted in complete cessation of her hemiplegic attacks. Six weeks after treatment was begun she had her first MRS study which revealed an abnormally high P_i, low PCr, high calculated free cytosolic ADP, and low PP (Table 1). Her attacks were completely controlled for one year and her motor language and academic performance

TABLE 1. *Results of phosphorus spectroscopy of muscle in three patients with AHC studied on two or three occasions over a 3-year period*

Examination	P_i (mM)	PCr (mM)	ADP (μM)	PP (M^{-1})
Patient 1				
1st	7.6	24.1	36	29
2nd	3.6	28.1	26	84
3rd	5.3	30.3	22	69
Patient 2				
1st	6.9	29.5	24	47
2nd	6.5	34.2	15	79
Patient 3				
1st	4.6	30.7	19	89
2nd	7.4	30.6	22	50
3rd	8.8	32.3	19	47
Normal control mean ± 1 SD	3.6 ± 0.48	32.6 ± 2.2	17 ± 4.7	145 ± 55
Patient mean and p (first exam)	6.4 ($p < 0.005$)	28.1 ($p < 0.05$)	26 ($p < 0.05$)	55 ($p < 0.01$)
Patient mean and p (all exams)	6.3 ($p < 0.005$)	30.4 ($p < 0.1$)	23 ($p < 0.1$)	62 ($p < 0.05$)

P_i, inorganic phosphate; PCr, phosphocreatine; ADP, adenosine phosphate; PP, phosphorylation potential.

improved substantially. A follow-up MRS performed at 5 years of age showed improvement when compared to the initial study. At 6 years of age she developed a flu-like illness and over the next 3 months had a recurrence of 10 attacks of hemiplegia. A third MRS study revealed some deterioration and decrease in the PCr to P_i ratio compared to the previous examination.

Patient 2

This 27-year-old woman was born after a normal pregnancy and delivery. At 3 months of age she started having episodes of rigidity, extension of the right arm, flushing, and apnea. At 7 months of age she developed episodes of flaccid hemiplegia involving one or both sides of the body occurring up to 5 times per day. Initially the attacks were associated with nystagmus, but this resolved. Prior to the attacks she would become upset and cry as if in pain. At 12 years of age she developed tonic clonic seizures. In recent years she has had intermittent bouts of status epilepticus (see Chapter 29). She now suffers from severe psychomotor retardation, microcephaly, hypotonia, and choreoathetosis with dystonic posturing of her arms. She walks with a semi-flexed, simian gait. In recent years she has been fairly stable. She receives valproic acid, phenytoin, and primidone. Her attacks of hemiplegia continue to occur about 4 times per month.

Her initial phosphorus MRS exam was performed at 26 years of age at a time when her seizure disorder was poorly controlled. This showed a moderately high P_i with borderline PCr, ADP, and PP. A follow-up study at a time when seizures were better controlled showed a slight improvement in energy state.

Proton MRS of periventricular brain revealed an NAA/CR relative resonance intensity ratio more than two standard deviations below the normal control mean on both examinations (Fig. 2). It did not show any abnormality in lactate concentration.

Patient 3

This 12-year-old girl was born of a normal pregnancy after a 72-hour home labor. At 3 months of age she had attacks of hyperventilation, tremor, hypertonicity, and staring occurring several times per day. At 7 months she developed episodes of lateral head and eye deviation and left dystonia. Multiple attacks of flaccid hemiparesis developed on either side of the body lasting from hours to days. These were provoked by excitement and bright lights and were relieved by sleep. Mild mental retardation, spastic hemiparesis, gait ataxia, tremor, and choreoathetosis have developed. In recent years she has had alternating hemiplegic attacks approximately 3 times per week. Flunarizine decreased their duration. Seizures have not been fully controlled when receiving clobazam and phenytoin, but have been brief and did not represent a severe problem. Choreoathetosis has progressed slowly.

Her initial phosphorus MRS was performed at age 8 years. This showed only a

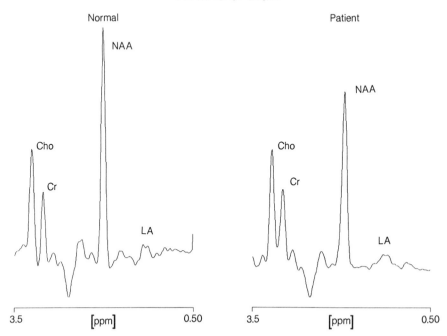

FIG. 2. Proton MR spectrum from a normal subject and patient 2. Note the low value of NAA/Cr.

minimal abnormality in PCr/P_i and PP. Subsequent examinations showed deterioration in the energy state of muscle.

DISCUSSION

Phosphorus MRS of muscle and proton MRS of brain reveal metabolic abnormalities in patients with AHC. The nature of the abnormalities, i.e., the low energy state of phosphate-containing metabolites of intermediary metabolism are consistent with mitochondrial dysfunction (1–3). This pattern of mitochondrial dysfunction involving asymptomatic muscle in patients with cerebral dysfunction is suggestive of a primary mitochondrial cytopathy (13). Certain features of AHC, such as dystonia, choreoathetosis, and precipitation by stress, are reminiscent of those of other recognized mitochondrial phenotypes and lend clinical support to the biochemical findings. The low NAA/Cr ratio reflects neuronal loss and damage that underlies the progressive cognitive impairment shown by the patients. We speculate that this neuronal loss and damage may be secondary to mitochondrial dysfunction.

The metabolic abnormality in muscle fluctuated over time to a greater extent than what is seen in normal muscle and the severity of the metabolic abnormality appeared to correlate with the clinical status of the patients. We have seen a similar phenomenon in patients with Leigh's disease in whom muscle spectra may be normal or almost normal when the patient is well and grossly abnormal during metabolic decompensation (14). MRS may thus be a useful surrogate marker for assessing the status of the disease and following the metabolic response to treatment.

We have seen abnormalities on MRS consistent with mitochondrial dysfunction in patients with a number of neurological disorders that have some features of AHC. A patient with pyruvate dehydrogenase deficiency and episodes of hemiplegia (see Chapter 20) had a severely impaired energy state of phosphate-containing metabolites in muscle and also an approximately fivefold increase in cerebral parenchymal lactate concentration. These abnormalities were much more severe than those in our patients with AHC. One of two patients with familial hemiplegic migraine (see Chapter 22), and one of two patients with benign familial nocturnal AHC (see Chapter 17) showed abnormalities in phosphorus spectra of muscle similar to those of patients with AHC. These patients may form part of an as yet ill-defined group of patients with fluctuating neurological dysfunction that may be related to mitochondrial dysfunction.

ACKNOWLEDGMENTS

The authors are grateful to Gilles Leroux and Andre Cormier for providing excellent technical support.

REFERENCES

1. Matthews PM, Allaire C, Shoubridge EA, Karpati G, Carpenter S, Arnold DL. In vivo muscle magnetic resonance spectroscopy in the clinical investigation of mitochondrial disease. *Neurology* 1991;41:114–120.
2. Arnold DL, Matthews PM, Radda GK. Metabolic recovery after exercise and the assessment of mitochondrial function in vivo in human skeletal muscle by means of ^{31}P NMR. *Magn Reson Med* 1984;1:307–315.
3. Arnold DL, Taylor DJ, Radda GK. Investigation of human mitochondrial myopathies by phosphorus magnetic resonance spectroscopy. *Ann Neurol* 1985;18:189–196.
4. Simmons ML, Frondoza CG, Coyle JT. Immunocytochemical localization of N-acetyl-aspartate with monoclonal antibodies. *Neuroscience* 1991;45:37–45.
5. Moffett JR, Namboodiri MM, Cangro CB, Neale JH. Immunohistochemical localization of N-acetylaspartate in rat brain. *Neuroreport* 1991;2:131–134.
6. Arnold DL, Silver K, Andermann F. Evidence for mitochondrial dysfunction in patients with alternating hemiplegia of childhood. *Ann Neurol* 1993;33:604–607.
7. Aicardi J. Alternating hemiplegia of childhood. *Int Pediatr* 1987;2:115–119.
8. de Beer R, van Ormondt D, Pijnappel WWF. Improved harmonic retrieval from noisy signals by invoking prior knowledge. In: Lacome JL, Chehikan A, Martin N, Malbos J, eds. *Signal processing IV: theories and applications.* Amsterdam: Elsevier; 1988:1283–1286.
9. Harris RC, Hultman E, Nordesjo L-O. Glycogen, glycolytic intermediates and high-energy phosphates determined in biopsy samples of musculus quadriceps femoris of man at rest. Methods and variance of values. *Scand J Clin Lab Invest* 1974;33:109–120.

10. Sjogaard G, Saltin B. Extra- and intracellular water spaces in muscles of man at rest and with dynamic exercise. *Am J Physiol* 1982;243:R271–R280.
11. Garlick PB, Radda GK, Seeley PJ. Studies of acidosis in the ischemic heart by phosphorus magnetic resonance. *Biochem J* 1979;184:547–554.
12. Heindel W, Bunke J, Glathe S, Steinbrich W, Mollevanger L. Combined ¹H-MR imaging and localized ³¹P-spectroscopy of intracranial tumors in 43 patients. *J Comput Assist Tomogr* 1988;12: 907–916.
13. Matthews PM, Berkovic SF, Shoubridge EA, et al. In vivo magnetic resonance spectroscopy of brain and muscle in a type of mitochondrial encephalomyopathy (MERRF). *Ann Neurol* 1991;29: 435–438.
14. Sylvain M, Mitchell GA, Shevell MI, et al. Muscle and brain magnetic resonance spectroscopy and imaging in children with Leigh's syndrome associated with cytochrome *c* oxidase deficiency: Dependence of findings on clinical status. *Ann Neurol* 1993;34:464.(abst).

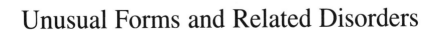

Unusual Forms and Related Disorders

Alternating Hemiplegia of Childhood, edited by
Frederick Andermann, Jean Aicardi, and Federico Vigevano,
Raven Press, Ltd., New York © 1995.

16

Autosomal Dominant Alternating Hemiplegia of Childhood

Mohamad A. Mikati, *Lorcan O'Tuama, and **Fernando Dangond

*Department of Neurology, and *Department of Radiology, Children's Hospital;
**Department of Neurology, Brigham and Women's Hospital, Harvard Medical School,
300 Longwood Avenue, Boston, MA 02115.*

We recently reported the first familial occurrence of alternating hemiplegia of child-hood (AHC) with the results of EEG, SPECT, and chromosomal investigations (Table 1) (1). Until that time AHC had been considered a nonfamilial syndrome. Other than a report of two identical twins being affected with the disorder, no truly familial cases had been noted since all the other approximately 30 cases in the literature had been sporadic (2,3). In this chapter the clinical characteristics and the laboratory investigations of the above family are presented. In addition to detailing the previously reported material about this family (1), we also report some further clinical details of this family and provide a synopsis of the results of a survey we performed on cases of AHC (2).

SURVEY RESULTS

Cases were ascertained through a call for patients announcement sent through the United States Child Neurology Society to all child neurologists who are members of that society (2). Physicians responding positively that they had patients with AHC were asked to provide summaries of their cases. In many instances telephone inter-views of the families by the author of this chapter were also performed. Thirty-seven cases from 23 states were initially ascertained. Thirty-seven percent were female and 67% were male. Mean current age was 9 years (range 1–42 years). The condition was frequently misdiagnosed as epilepsy, and several months or years usually elapsed before the correct diagnosis was usually made. Some patients were seen by as many as seven neurologists before the correct diagnosis was made. Re-ported symptoms that were invariably present included hemiplegia episodes and extrapyramidal symptoms in the form of dystonic spells and/or choreoathetosis. Developmental delay was present in all except for possibly one patient. The severity

TABLE 1. *Comparison of the sporadic and autosomal dominant cases of AHC*

Symptom	Sporadic AHC cases	Autosomal dominant AHC cases
Onset<18 months	+	+
Hemiplegia spells	+	+
Double hemiplegia spells	+	+
Dystonic spells	+	+
Choreoathetosis	+	+
Paroxysmal oculomotor abnormalities	+	+
Autonomic disturbances	+	+
Developmental retardation	+	+
Remission in sleep	+	+

of the delay was usually moderate but it varied from very mild to very severe. Other symptoms included episodes of double hemiplegia, eye movement abnormalities, and autonomic dysfunction. Common manifestations also included seizures and family history of migraine. Antiepileptic drugs, as a rule were not helpful although a rare case may have responded to benzodiazepines when given on a chronic basis or acutely for an attack. Most patients received and had partially responded to flunarizine treatment. The clinical course of the disorder generally showed persistence of the symptoms with fluctuation and at times some progression was evident. Since reviewing the above 37 cases, 14 additional cases from the United States and one from Saudi Arabia have also come to our attention. These cases also fitted the above profile. Because of ascertainment bias based on the fact that neurologists will report cases consistent with the preset and previously known criteria of the disease (3), it is difficult to truly determine at this stage the full significance of some of the above data, such as the significance and true incidence of the family history of migraine. However, none of the above cases or of any of those reported previously in the literature (other than ours), gave a true family history of alternating hemiplegia.

CASE HISTORIES

The Proband

Ed. A. was the product of a full term pregnancy and was delivered by C-section for failure of labor to progress. Birth weight was 8 lb and there was no neonatal distress. Early development was within normal limits. He sat at 5 months, stood at 8 months, and spoke using single words at 10 months. However, he did not walk independently until 23 months. His history consisted of the following:

1. He was evaluated at the age of 2 months because of an episode of left arm and left leg stiffening with deviation of the eyes. An EEG showed right occipital sharp waves and CT scan revealed slight ventricular dilatation and widening of

the subarachnoid space. He was started on phenobarbital. During the next several months, he was seen repeatedly for seizures, each lasting 5–10 minutes, consisting of "generalized shaking of all four extremities," or of left-sided tonic-clonic movements.

2. At about the age of 6 months, distinct and independent 5–10 minute episodes of isolated unilateral (right-sided) weakness with eye deviation to the left were described but, at the time, were presumed to represent postictal paralysis of unwitnessed left hemisphere focal seizures. A repeat EEG at the age of 12 months was normal. There was poor control of the hemiplegic spells. Phenytoin was added.

3. At the age of 14 months the patient was witnessed in the hospital to have serial episodes of generalized hypotonia and limpness while fully awake and while being able to look at his mother and recognize her. Anticonvulsant levels during these spells were therapeutic. Neuropsychological testing revealed a normal Bayley score.

4. At age 18 months, the proband was evaluated for a three-day history of inability to move the right arm without any preceding focal or generalized seizure activity. Examination showed a completely flaccid areflexic paralysis of the right upper extremity with no long tract or sensory signs. Radiographs of the right shoulder, forearm, and elbow were negative. EMG/nerve conduction studies of the right arm were negative. The weakness improved spontaneously and gradually. It completely resolved within one week.

5. Over the next several years the patient continued to have (a) rare generalized tonic-clonic seizures, (b) occasional left- or right-sided tonic posturing, and (c) distinct episodes of focal or generalized hypotonia. During this period, he was receiving phenobarbital or dilantin alone or in combination. At age 5 years, sodium valproate was added with no real improvement of the hemiplegic episodes.

At 6 years of age the patient was having daily hemiplegic or quadriplegic spells each lasting 5–20 minutes, several of which were reported to be precipitated by emotional stress. At that time he was referred to us with the presumptive diagnosis of intractable epilepsy. On admission to our hospital valproate and phenobarbital concentrations were 73 and 21 µg/dl, respectively. During an inpatient admission he underwent continuous long-term EEG monitoring. The EEG failed to reveal any changes during or after these episodes (see below). Blood chemistry, electromyography, nerve conduction studies, lactate, pyruvate, serum amino acid chromatography, and urinary 24-hour organic acid chromatography were all normal. Electron and light microscopy of the right quadriceps muscle biopsy showed mild variation in fiber diameter but no ragged red fibers or mitochondrial abnormalities. A neuropsychological evaluation revealed significant developmental delay with an overall functional level and a Stanford-Binet score between 2 and 3 years of age. The patient was tapered off all antiepileptic drugs without any increase in the frequency of his spells. The tonic-clonic seizures which were last noted at 5 years of age never recurred. On follow-up over the next 3 years the patient continued to have almost daily attacks of alternating hemiplegia when not receiving flunarizine treatment (see below). The attacks were not associated with any apparent headaches and he was not having any tonic-clonic seizures. In between the attacks the choreoathetosis and dystonic posturing became progressively more prominent, almost continuous, and frequently increased upon attempted movements. Most of the choreoathetosis and posturing involved the upper extremities although the face, lower extremities, and trunk were also involved.

Father (II, 2)

Eli. A. is now a 42-year-old man who was first evaluated by us at the age of 39 years. He was reported to have had unilateral or bilateral episodes of arm and/or leg paralysis since the first year of life. These episodes were often precipitated by emotional stress and were initially not associated with headaches or mental status changes. Trials of phenytoin and of multiple other antiepileptic drugs had been unsuccessful in controlling these spells. In addition, the patient also had much less frequent generalized tonic-clonic seizures. His workup had included a normal CT scan with and without contrast, normal electrolytes, calcium, magnesium, glucose, and liver function tests. His electroencephalogram showed right temporal slowing. The father's exam during a left hemiplegic attack showed unilateral upper and lower extremity hemiplegia, increased tone and hyperreflexia with an otherwise normal neurologic exam. In between the attacks his exam showed athetoid movements of the upper extremities, posturing of the left upper extremity, and a slightly wide-based ataxic gait. He had five siblings (one sister) only one of whom (a male) was affected with AHC. The history and findings of that sibling are described below.

Uncle (II, 1)

The uncle gave a history of unilateral and at times bilateral paroxysmal episodes of arm and/or leg weakness usually lasting several minutes to hours but on certain rare occasions for as long as several weeks. He first came to our attention during the proband's hospitalization. The events occasionally followed emotional stress and had begun by the age of 3 years. The patient was observed during an episode of right hemiplegia. This episode progressed into almost complete quadriplegia that lasted for 45 minutes. During that period he was unable to speak but mental status examination, performed by head nods/yes-no questioning, was normal. Respiration was not compromised. There was bilateral nasolabial fold flattening, and he had decreased facial movements. His gag was present and cranial nerve examination was otherwise normal. There was complete flaccid paralysis of his extremities except for slight movement of the right deltoid. There was normal position and pinprick sensation. Reflexes were absent except for 1 + right triceps and biceps. Plantar responses were flexor. After 45 minutes of complete quadriplegia, the left side gradually recovered to full strength within a period of 10 minutes. The right hemiparesis, however, persisted for several days after that. During the above attack, ammonia, calcium, magnesium, phosphorus, glucose, and serum electrolytes were all normal.

Symptomatic Brother (III, 3)

Elv. A. was a 3-year-old boy who had been investigated for developmental delay during his first year of life but a positive diagnosis could not be established. Two months after the proband's admission, Elv. A. presented with a history of gait difficulty of one day's duration. He had no prior history of seizures or hemiplegic attacks. On examination, he was noted to be dragging the left leg and to have decreased spontaneous movements of the left arm. Tendon reflexes were 2+ throughout and plantar responses were flexor. The rest of the neurologic examination was normal. Computerized cranial tomography and a spinal tap were normal. Electrolytes, glucose, calcium, magnesium, phosphorus, CBC, platelet count, clotting time, serum viscosity, lactate, protein C, protein S, antithrombin III, and EEG were all within normal limits. His hemiplegia resolved over 24 hours and he was discharged home. Over the next 2 years he continued to develop episodes of alternating hemiplegia at a rate of one attack every few weeks. On follow-up 2½ years later his MRI was normal and most of his attacks were reported to have become dystonic rather than hemiplegic in nature.

Asymptomatic Brother (III, 2)

This was a 6-year-old boy reported to have learning disability but who had not had episodes of alternating hemiplegia. He had a normal neurological examination. Further testing of this child was not possible.

Paternal Grandmother (I, 2)

The paternal grandmother, who was deceased at the time this family came to our attention, was reported to have had similar hemi and/or quadriplegic attacks starting in early childhood and subsiding in her forties.

LABORATORY INVESTIGATIONS

Karyotype

Karyotyping with QFQ and GTG banding of metaphase cells was performed on the proband, his siblings, mother, father, and uncle. The analysis was performed at least at the 400 band level of resolution. In all the subjects except for sibling (III, 2) karyotyping was performed on cultured peripheral blood lymphocytes. In sibling (III, 2) lymphocyte cultures failed to grow and thus his karyotype was performed on fibroblasts grown from skin biopsy.

Restriction Fragment Length Polymorphism (RFLP) Linkage Analysis

The methods used were described in detail in previous publications (1,4–12). DNA was extracted from lymphoblastoid lines or whole blood as previously described (4). Samples of DNA (5–10μg) were digested to completion with restriction enzymes according to manufacturers' instructions. Electrophoresis was carried out routinely in 0.8% agarose gels at 70–90 V for 16 hours. DNA fragments were blotted onto Genetran nylon membranes (Plasco, Woburn, MA) by the method of Southern. Filters were prehybridized and hybridized in 0.3% sodium dodecyl sulfate, $1 \times$ Denhardt's solution, $6 \times$ sodium chloride/sodium citrate (SSC) containing salmon sperm DNA at 65°C; washed at 65°C in decreasing concentrations of SSC to $0.5 \times$, and exposed to x-ray film. Lymphoblastoid lines were available on the proband, both parents, and both siblings of the family being studied. DNA probes were labeled with [^{32}P]dATP (3,000 Ci/mmol; Amersham, Arlington Heights, IL) by random oligonucleotide priming (5).

The following polymorphic marker probes were used (6–12): random VNTR locus *D9S* (EFD 61.3) on chromosome 9 q34-qter; (GT)n polymorphism for locus *GSN* on 9 q32-34, (GT)n polymorphism for locus *ASS* on 9q34-qter; and (GT)n polymorphism for locus *D3S270* on 3 p26 (S. Klauck and B. Seizinger, *unpublished data* 1992). (GT)n polymorphisms were resolved using the polymerase chain reaction (PCR) to amplify the repeat containing regions. Reaction volumes were 10 μl and contained 0.2 mM dATP, dCTP, dTTP; 2.5 μmdGTP; 4 ng each of oligonucleotide primer pairs; 0.08 μl 32-P dGTP (3,000 mCi/ml); 0.05 μl Taq polymerase and $1 \times$ reaction buffer (Perkin-Elmer Cetus). Thermal controller settings were 94° C for 1.5 min; 25 cycles of 94° C for 1 min, 55° C for 1 min, and 72° C for 10 min. Amplified products were analyzed as described in Kwiatkowski et al (10).

Single Photon Emission Tomography (SPECT)

SPECT scanning was performed as described previously (1,13). Patients III,1, the proband and III,3 were investigated in the asymptomatic state. Patient III,1 had the SPECT scan repeated at the time of complete right upper and lower extremity hemiplegia with preservation of consciousness, normal speech, normal visual fields, and intact sensations. Patient III,3 had a second interictal scan at the age of 6 years. All studies were read independently by three observers without a prior knowledge of the clinical facts. A dose of 5 mCi was used in both patients. SPECT acquisition and analysis was obtained using a rotating gamma camera (Orbiter; Siemens Medical Systems, Inc., Hoffman Estates, IL) 30 degree slant hole collimator, with transaxial resolution (full width at half maximum) of 14 mm. Tomographic imaging began at 30–60 minutes and continued for 45–60 minutes, using an acquisition time of 60 seconds per angle, and a 64-voxel-matrix. Image reconstruction and analysis was performed by an ADAC computer (ADAC Laboratories, San Jose, CA). Axial, coronal, and sagittal projections were displayed, and reviewed for analysis.

EEG

Long-term monitoring using 18 channels and the 10/20 system was performed on our proband. Split screen and continuous video recordings were performed during part of the monitoring and captured hemiplegic spells.

Therapy

Antiepileptic drug therapy with phenobarbital, phenytoin, and valproic acid was attempted in the proband, his father, and his uncle, but was not successful despite therapeutic levels. The proband also failed a trial of nimodipine. The father in addition had received diazepam and carbamazepine. There was no response of the alternating hemiplegia episodes to any of these medications. The proband could be tapered off all antiepileptic medications at the age of 6 years without recurrence of any of his epileptic seizures. When evaluated, the father was taking diazepam erratically and had not experienced any seizures for about 4 years. The proband and his symptomatic brother were both started, in a single blinded fashion, on flunarizine. Flunarizine is a calcium channel blocker that has been reported to reduce the frequency and severity of hemiplegic attacks in some patients with alternating hemiplegia (14,15). Flunarizine concentrations were measured by a standardized HPLC technique. The daily dose was 0.24 mg/kg (5 mg) per day for the proband and 0.15 mg/kg per day (5 mg 3 times per week) for his brother. The frequency of the attacks was recorded for 2 months before and 4 months after the initiation of therapy.

RESULTS

Karyotype

The proband and both of his brothers, his father, and his uncle had a balanced 46, XY,t(3:9)(p26;q34) karyotype. The asymptomatic mother had a normal 46,XX karyotype.

Linkage Analysis Results

Analysis using the *GSN* probe was not useful because the father was homozygous for that polymorphic marker. Both parents were heterozygous for the *D9S*, *ASS*, and the *D3S270* polymorphic markers. The patterns for these markers are summarized in Fig. 1. These results confirmed the karyotype results and indicated that the *ASS* and *EFD* sites were segregating with the t(3;9)(p26;q34) translocation.

SPECT

The SPECT scan performed on the proband during right hemiplegia did not show any significant change from the one performed during the asymptomatic period (Fig. 2). The resolution of SPECT scanning, however, was not sufficient to rule out minor changes in perfusion such as those involving very restricted regions of the cortex, basal ganglia, internal capsule, and/or deeper brainstem structures. In the other patient (III,3) an initial "interictal" SPECT was normal but a repeat scan 16 months later showed relatively decreased perfusion involving the left temporoparietal areas.

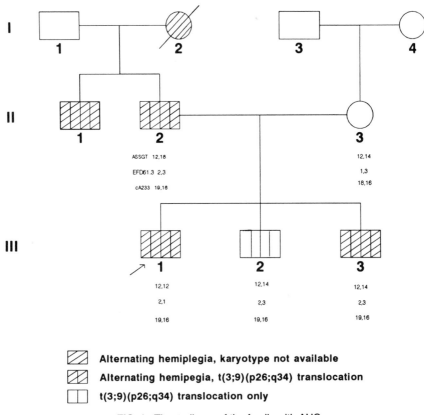

FIG. 1. The pedigree of the family with AHC.

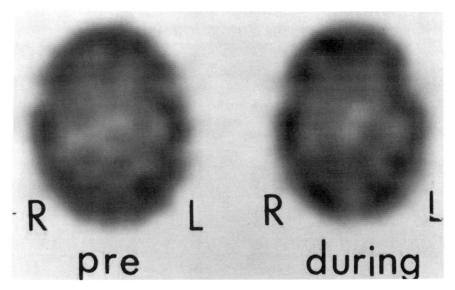

FIG. 2. HMPAO SPECT images from our proband before and during a right hemiplegic attack. The images display transaxial slices at the level of the lower parietal lobes.

EEG

During his long-term monitoring the proband manifested hemiplegic attacks, unilateral or bilateral choreoathetosis, and less frequent dystonic posturing of the extremities. Several spells characterized by acute onset of generalized or unilateral floppiness and paralysis were recorded. During the quadriplegic attacks cranial nerves were usually intact and the patient turned to voice and moaned. He grimaced to pinprick in all four extremities and was areflexic. Plantar responses were flexor. During the attacks of partial or complete unilateral upper and lower extremity flaccid hemiplegia there was some slurring of speech but no alteration of consciousness, language, or cranial nerve function. On the hemiplegic side deep tendon reflexes were usually suppressed and the plantar response was variable. These attacks lasted up to 45 minutes and after them the patient quickly returned to baseline manifesting his mild ataxia and prominent choreoathetoid movements in the upper extremities. The EEG was normal throughout all these episodes. In particular, during complete hemiplegia or quadriplegia, the EEG showed no changes with persistence of normal activity including mu. Complete blocking of mu was not noted upon the request to move the hemiplegic side (Fig. 3).

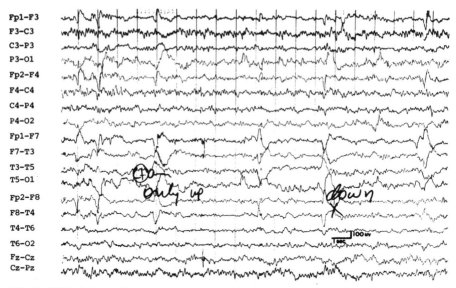

FIG. 3. EEG of the proband during an attack of complete right-sided hemiplegia showing a normal background and a normal central mu rhythm. The patient is asked to raise his arms and in response he is able to raise only his left arm with blocking of the mu rhythm on the right side. The mu rhythm on the left side persists and manifests only minimal attenuation during that period.

Therapy

Baseline hemiplegic attack frequency (during the 2 months preceding onset of flunarizine therapy) was 5.8 and 3.4 attacks per week in the proband and in his brother, respectively. During the 4 months of single-blinded therapy there was an initial gradual (first month) and then a sustained decrease in the frequency of their hemiplegic attacks. During these 4 months the frequency of the attacks was 1.6 and 0.3 attacks per week, respectively. This represented a 72% and 91% decrease in attack rate. The severity and duration of attacks were also decreased. Trough flunarizine concentrations were obtained on both patients after 3 months of therapy and these were 28.9 and 6.6 μg/ml for the proband and his brother, respectively.

DISCUSSION

Clinical Features

The syndrome of AHC was first described in 1971 (16). More recently the boundaries of the syndrome were defined by Aicardi (3,17). Criteria for diagnosis by Aicardi include:

1. Onset before 18 months of age.
2. Repeated bouts of hemiplegia of varying intensity involving both sides of the body.
3. Other paroxysmal phenomena including tonic spells, dystonic posturing, choreoathetoid movements, nystagmus, or other ocular abnormalities, and autonomic disturbances during and between hemiplegic attacks.
4. Evidence of mental and neurologic deficits with a progressive course.

Our index patient and all other affected family members satisfy the above criteria. The onset of hemiplegic attacks was delayed till the age of 3 years in the proband's sibling (III,3). However this patient's developmental delay, which is one of the manifestations of this syndrome, was evident before his first birthday. Hemiplegic attacks without preceding seizure activity were noted in the proband during the first year of life. Intermittent choreoathetoid movements and ataxia prompted a negative workup for Wilson's disease, metachromatic leukodystrophy, and abetalipoproteinemia. Pyruvate decarboxylase deficiency, porphyria and ornithine transcarbamylase deficiency, were also ruled out. Finally, developmental and cognitive testing illustrated progressive intellectual decline associated with this disorder. Laboratory, electrophysiologic, radiographic, and muscle biopsy studies further confirmed the clinical diagnosis by excluding other possible causes of acute hemiplegia. Serial CT and MRI scans, while showing mild atrophy, revealed no evidence of stroke or other neurodegenerative diseases such as Schilder's disease or mitochondrial encephalomyopathy. The lack of occurrence of permanent focal deficits or strokes and the clinical course of the disorder in the proband and in other family members did not justify performing an arteriogram. Embolic phenomena from the heart are unlikely, based on the clinical course and the negative echocardiographic examinations.

A number of conditions may have presentations that can mimic aspects of AHC. These conditions include moyamoya disease (18,19), paroxysmal dystonia, periodic paralysis, hemiplegic migraine, and epilepsy. In paroxysmal dystonia, which begins in early life and can be familial, there is sudden loss of motor control in the arms and legs (20). However in this syndrome the loss of motor control is characterized by flexion dystonia, not flaccid weakness as was observed. The familial periodic paralyses are associated with episodic bouts of generalized (rather than unilateral) weakness. During an attack, muscle is unexcitable by EMG stimulation. Abnormalities of serum levels of potassium are usually found. The proband and his uncle had normal serum potassium levels during their attacks. Electromyographic and nerve conduction examinations were normal in the proband during an attack. Migraine may also be familial and may result in extremity weakness (21,22). It may not necessarily be accompanied by headache. However, migraines are not associated with progressive cognitive decline, choreiform movements, or dystonic posturing. The initial description of patients with AHC referred to those patients as cases of complicated migraine. However, it is now clear they have a distinct, though possibly related, clinical entity.

The original premise in our proband was that the episodic hemiplegic attacks were seizure phenomena. Our patients do not fit any of the known familial epileptic syndromes (23–25). During the attacks he showed no changes on EEG. Inhibitory seizures may cause hemiparesis. However, these seizures are associated with EEG changes, they respond to antiepileptic medications, and they do not manifest, the natural history exhibited by our patients (26).

The hemiplegic attacks of AHC do not satisfy any of these criteria and thus can not be considered classic epileptic seizures. Dystonic seizures can originate from the frontal lobe, but electroencephalographic changes should accompany them (27). This was not the case in our patients. Epileptic seizures, however, are part of the symptoms of AHC. This can make establishing the diagnosis of AHC particularly difficult. In our family the proband, his father, and the paternal uncle had definite prior focal and/or generalized tonic-clonic seizures in addition to their hemiplegic spells. All three are no longer receiving maintenance anticonvulsant therapy and while they continue to suffer from hemiplegic episodes, they do not complain of their previously described tonic-clonic seizures. Despite normal or mildly abnormal interictal EEGs and despite the lack of postictal confusion, each of the three affected patients described above were initially presumed to have "refractory epilepsy." Our patients thus illustrate the importance of being aware of this syndrome in order to be able to appropriately identify, hopefully early, those patients who are affected by it.

Inheritance

In this family autosomal dominant inheritance is almost certainly demonstrated since the syndrome has appeared in three generations and both sexes were affected. Although both the apparently related disorders, epilepsy and migraine, are frequently familial and may exhibit autosomal dominant inheritance (21–25), our patients do not fit any of the known migrainous or epileptic syndromes.

The possible association with (t3;9)(p26;q34) translocation is intriguing. The presence of this translocation in both the father, the uncle, and in the two affected siblings raises the question whether the gene predisposing to alternating hemiplegia may not be located on the short arm of chromosome 3 or the long arm of chromosome 9 close to where the translocation breakpoint occurs. Subject (III,2) however, had the translocation but did not manifest alternating hemiplegia. Several potential explanations for this observation exist:

1. The translocation is incidental and is not related to the alternating hemiplegia.
2. The translocation and the hemiplegia are related and are segregating together, however, there is variable penetrance of alternating hemiplegia. Consequently the subject III, 2 may be carrying the gene defect for alternating hemiplegia but is not manifesting the full disorder yet. This hypothesis is supported by the fact that this disorder manifested a variable degree of severity and of age of onset in

different members of the family. It is thus possible that the sibling (III,2) who was reported to have a significant learning disability may still develop alternating hemiplegia. His learning disability may be a minor manifestation of the phenotype which does include developmental delay. Developmental delay in the other two affected siblings did manifest with school difficulty.

3. The translocation and the alternating hemiplegia are related and segregating together in the father, the uncle, and the two affected siblings; however, in the unaffected sibling there has been a very small chromosomal rearrangement, causing the translocation and the alternating hemiplegia gene to segregate independently. Thus this child may have inherited the translocation without inheriting the defective gene associated with alternating hemiplegia. This last hypothesis is highly unlikely and is not supported by the results of our RFLP analysis.

We believe that our data suggest that the alternating hemiplegia gene in our family may be located on 3p or 9q. Karyotyping and linkage studies on other patients with AHC particularly those that may be familial should be performed in order to further investigate this possibility. It is intriguing that the dominantly acting gene for idiopathic paroxysmal torsion dystonia has been located on chromosome 9q32–34 (4,28) and that our patients manifested prominent choreoathetosis as well as dystonia.

Pathophysiology

The pathophysiology of alternating hemiplegia remains obscure. In our proband, the lack of significant electroencephalographic or SPECT changes during the attacks as well as the clinical manifestations argue against widespread cortical hemispherical involvement. AHC patients typically do not manifest any aphasia, visual field defects, or sensory changes during their attacks. This tends to favor involvement of one of the following:

1. A very restricted area of the frontal motor strip,
2. Internal capsule,
3. Cerebral peduncles or corticospinal tract
4. The basal ganglia.

Involvement of areas supplied by the penetrating arteries such as the lenticulostriates is a plausible hypothesis. This would be consistent with the symptoms manifested by our patients and with their electrophysiologic findings. The ocular motor and autonomic symptoms that are also occasionally noted during the attacks may suggest additional brainstem and/or hypothalamic involvement. Basal ganglia involvement is indirectly supported by the extrapyramidal symptoms these patients manifest in between the hemiplegic attacks.

Investigations of blood flow changes in alternating hemiplegia during attacks have revealed apparently contradictory results. A number of investigators have reported ischemic focal changes in the hemisphere contralateral to the hemiplegia, some found no significant changes, and yet others described increased blood flow (29–36):

1. Blood flow studies with the ^{133}XE inhalation method in one patient with alternating hemiplegia (29) and with SPECT (30) showed *decreased* blood flow in the contralateral hemisphere. Using carotid Doppler, Aicardi (3) studied three patients during and between attacks. In two of the three patients there was no decrease in the carotid blood flow or velocity on the side opposite to the hemiplegia. In the third there was only a moderate decrease in velocity and flow.
2. Kanazawa and associates (32) reported that the HMPAO SPECT studies during alternating hemiplegia attacks of their patient showed *hyper*perfusion in the contralateral hemisphere. They considered this as evidence favoring the hypothesis that alternating hemiplegia is an atypical manifestation of epilepsy despite the lack of focal or epileptic ictal abnormalities.
3. Another report (33) was unclear as to whether there was hyperperfusion of the contralateral hemisphere.
4. Interictal studies measuring cerebral blood flow by SPECT and cerebral metabolic rate by PET reported an interictal decrease in cerebral blood flow and metabolism (33–36). This may not be inconsistent with the diffuse encephalopathy these patients have. One potential explanation for these apparently contradictory results is that there may be sequential changes in blood flow during the hemiplegic spells.

   In our proband there was no significant change in the SPECT scan during a hemiplegic spell. The significance of the relatively decreased perfusion involving the left temporoparietal lobe in patient III,3 in his second "asymptomatic" scan is not clear. The explanation of this finding cannot be related plausibly to a manifestation of epilepsy-related changes, since the patient had never experienced any epileptic seizures. He also had not experienced any clinical events for 12 hours before the study. No structural changes were noted on his MRI scan to account for the abnormal areas of tracer distribution. It is possible that the SPECT changes may indicate a subclinical dysfunction related to the diffuse and slowly progressive encephalopathy these patients have. While interpreting the apparently contradictory SPECT results it is important to note that SPECT imaging may be capable of showing areas of dysfunction within the cortex at sites that are transsynaptically connected with the basal ganglia. Such findings might explain at least in part the cortical perfusion changes noted in our second patient, as well as in some of the studies cited above.

   EEG studies have repeatedly failed to show epileptiform activity during hemiplegic attacks, but have otherwise been somewhat inconsistent:

1. Dalla Bernardina and associates (37) found focal EEG changes *contralateral* to the hemiplegia in 3/3 patients.

2. Hosking and associates (38) performed EEG studies on six patients during the attacks and in between them. When slow wave abnormalities were seen, these were diffuse and did not lateralize either during an attack or between attacks. Aicardi (3) also did *not* find any contralateral epileptic or focal EEG changes during hemiplegic attacks in his patients. All these findings suggest that either (a) there is heterogeneity in the pathogenesis of alternating hemiplegia and different authors are investigating different groups of patients each with a similar presentation but with a distinct pathophysiology, or (more likely) (b) the pathophysiology, as suggested by our data, does not necessarily have to involve major cortical structures. It may be predominantly restricted to small cortical and/or subcortical regions that are too small to be consistently and adequately assessed by the available noninvasive EEG and blood flow measurement techniques.

In the past the hemiplegic spells have been considered to be either secondary to migrainous type vasospasm or to seizure activity. There is conflicting evidence, reviewed above, that supports and argues against each of these two hypotheses. In our opinion it is difficult, though not impossible, to conceive of vasospasm as the only or the primary, problem causing all of the symptoms seen in AHC. We also believe that Todd's paralysis or inhibitory seizures do not provide a completely satisfactory explanation for the hemiplegic spells. To account for the at times frequent occurrence of quadriplegia with preservation of consciousness and for the lack of sensory symptoms during the attacks, one would have to assume a prolonged predominantly mesial and/or bilateral symmetrical involvement of very restricted areas of the frontal lobes without spread of the seizure discharges to any other area of the brain during these episodes. This and the EEG and SPECT findings discussed above make the seizure hypothesis less likely in our opinion.

In trying to formulate a hypothesis for explaining the pathogenesis of alternating hemiplegia, we believe there are several important observations that need to be clarified:

1. These patients have mild diffuse and at times focal cortical involvement. This is shown by the developmental delay and regression seen in all patients, as well as by the mild cortical atrophy and the epileptic seizures seen in some. This is also evidenced by the SPECT and EEG abnormalities.
2. There is evidence of subcortical involvement. The patients have significant extrapyramidal and ocular movement abnormalities between and during the attacks, respectively. They also have prominent autonomic abnormalities during attacks. The hypothesis presented below takes into account all these factors.

At present there is not enough evidence to establish a definitive mechanism for AHC. However we would like to propose a hypothesis that may be consistent with the currently available observations. It is possible that AHC is caused by a defect in the energy generation system (e.g., mitochondrial). Such an abnormality could presumably cause a diffuse encephalopathy with cortical involvement (as manifested by developmental delay) and with basal ganglia involvement (as evidenced by the extrapyramidal symptoms). Intermittent exacerbations in such a defect, possibly with secondary localized vasoprasm, may be responsible for the intermittent episodes of hemiplegia. Potential areas involved in the generation of the hemiplegia could include one or more of the following regions: frontal lobe, basal ganglia, internal capsule, brainstem, and at times possibly the entire affected cerebral hemisphere. Concurrent involvement of one or more of these areas would explain the occurrence of autonomic and ocular movement abnormalities during the hemiplegic spells. Epileptic seizures which do occur in some AHC patients could thus develop due to the cortical pathology that may result from such a defect. The MELAS and the MERRF syndromes manifest somewhat similar clinical profiles with a diffuse encephalopathy which is associated with intermittent focal symptoms and with seizures (42). However as Aicardi argues (3) the details of the clinical picture of AHC are significantly different. Additionally the negative muscle biopsy and the normal lactate and pyruvate levels in our patients did not support this hypothesis. Hence, if AHC is in fact one of the mitochondrial diseases then it must represent a very unusual form of this group of disorders. Because some patients with mitochondrial encephalopathies may have negative muscle biopsies and normal serum lactate and pyruvate levels we believe that our hypothesis continues to be attractive and needs to be investigated further.

Therapy

Flunarizine was effective in reducing the frequency of AHC spells in our patients. Whereas prior open-labeled reports have described response of alternating hemiplegia to flunarizine therapy, none of those studies reported serum concentrations of this medication (14,15,43,44). Flunarizine is primarily a smooth muscle relaxant which is effective in migraine prophylaxis (45). Although it does have some antiepileptic drug activity, we believe that the response to flunarizine treatment and the lack of improvement during traditional antiepileptic drug therapy provide support for the hypothesis that the direct causes responsible for the hemiplegic attacks involve predominantly neurovascular or metabolic rather than epileptic mechanisms.

SUMMARY

This chapter describes the familial occurrence of AHC in one family in whom the disorder was inherited as an autosomal dominant syndrome. Review of the cases described in the literature, and of approximately 60 cases ascertained through a survey of child neurologists in the United States revealed no other clearly familial cases. In the family we describe, two of three brothers, the father, an uncle, and the paternal grandmother were affected. The disorder was first recognized in the older 9-year-old brother when he presented with developmental retardation, rare tonic-clonic seizures, and frequent episodes of flaccid alternating hemiplegia that had been presumed to represent postictal paralysis. The hemiplegic spells, which started in the first year of life, did not respond to multiple antiepileptic agents. Between attacks there was choreoathetosis and dystonic posturing. Investigations included negative CT, metabolic, and coagulation studies. EEG and HMPAO SPECT scanning failed to reveal any significant slowing or major changes in cortical perfusion, respectively, during hemiplegia as compared to non-hemiplegic periods. Both the 9-year-old patient and his affected brother were treated with, and responded to, flunarizine therapy. Both had a greater than 70% decrease in attack frequency. Flunarizine trough serum concentrations were 28.9 and 6.6 µg/ml, respectively. Karyotype revealed a balanced reciprocal translocation 46, XY, t(3;9)(p26; q34) in the two affected brothers, the father, the affected uncle, and in one apparently unaffected sibling. The paternal grandmother could not be tested, while the asymptomatic mother had a normal karyotype. RFLP linkage analysis demonstrated that the markers contiguous to the translocation break point were segregating with the translocation.

ACKNOWLEDGMENT

Supported in part by the Wark Epilepsy Research Fund.

REFERENCES

1. Mikati MA, Maguire H, Barlow CF, et al. A syndrome of autosomal dominant alternating hemiplegia: Clinical presentation mimicking intractable epilepsy; chromosomal studies; and physiologic investigations. *Neurology* 1992;42:2251–2257.
2. Mikati MA, The United States Alternating Hemiplegia Group. Alternating hemiplegia of childhood: The United States cases. *Ann Neurol* 1992;32:451.
3. Aicardi J. Alternating hemiplegia of childhood. *Int Pediatr* 1987;2:115–119.
4. Kramer PL, deLeon D, Ozelius L, et al. Dystonia gene in Ashkenazi Jewish population is located on chromosome 9q32–34. *Ann Neurol* 1990;27:114–120.
5. Feinberg AP, Vogelstein B. Addendum to "A technique for radiolabeling DNA restriction endonuclease fragments to high specific activity." *Anal Biochem* 1984;137:266–267.
6. Lathrop M, Nakamura Y, O'Connell P, Leppert M, Woodard S, Lalouel JM, White R. A mapped set of genetic markers for human chromosome 9. *Genomics* 1988;3:361–366.
7. Kwiatkowski DJ, Westbrook, CA, Bruns GAB, Morton CC. Localization of gelsolin proximal to *ABL* on chromosome 9. *Am J Hum Genet* 1988;42:565–572
8. Kwiatowski DJ, Ozelius L, Schuback D, et al. The gelsolin cDNA clone from 9q34–34 identifies BclI and stuI RFLPs. *Nucleic Acids Res* 1989;17:4425.
9. Kwiatkowski DJ, Perman S. GTn dinucleotide repeat polymorphism within the *GSN* locus. *Nucleic Acids Res* 1991;19:4967.
10. Kwiatkowski DJ, Nygaard TG, Schuback DE, et al. Identification of a highly polymorphic microsatellite VNTR within the argininosuccinate synthetase locus: exclusion of the dystonia gene on 9q32–34 as the cause of dopa-responsive dystonia in a large kindred. *Am J Hum Gen* 1991;48:121–128.
11. Northrop H, Lathrop GM, Ying S-L, et al. Multilocus linkage analysis with a human argininosuccinate synthetase gene. *Genomics* 1989;5:442–444.
12. Beaudet AL, SU TS, O'Brien WE, et al. Dispersion of argininosuccinate-synthetase-like human genes to multiple autosome and the X chromosome. *Cell* 1982;30:287–293.

13. O'Tuama LA, Janicek M, Barnes PD, Scott RM, et al. 201-Tl/^{99m}Tc-HMPAO SPECT imaging of treated childhood brain tumors. *Pediatric Neurology* 1991;7:4:249–257.
14. Casaer P. Flunarizine in alternating hemiplegia childhood. An international study in 12 children. *Neuropediatrics* 1987;18:191–195.
15. Casaer P, Azou M. Flunarizine in alternating hemiplegia in childhood (Letter). *Lancet* 1984;2:579.
16. Verret S, Steele J. Alternating hemiplegia in childhood: A report of eight patients with complicated migraine beginning in infancy. *Pediatrics* 1971;47:675–680.
17. Krägeloh, I, Aicardi, J. Alternating hemiplegia in infants: Report of five cases. *Dev Med Child Neurol* 1980;22:784–791.
18. Carlson CB, Harvey FH, Loop J. Progressive alternating hemiplegia in early childhood and basal arterial stenosis and telangiectasia (moyamoya syndrome). *Neurology* 1973;23:734–44.
19. Cornelio-Nieto JO, Davila-Gutierrez G, Ferreyro-Irigoyen R, Alcala H. Acute hemiplegia in childhood and alternating hemiconvulsions secondary to Moya-Moya disease. Report of a case associated with Down's syndrome. *Bol Med Hosp Infant Mex* 1990;47:39–42.
20. Lance J. Familial paroxysmal dystonic choreoathetosis and its differentiation from related syndromes. *Ann Neurol* 1977;2:285–293.
21. Ohta M, Araki S, Kuroiwa Y. Familial occurrence of migraine with a hemiplegic syndrome and cerebellar manifestations. *Neurology* 1967;17:813–817.
22. Young GF, Leonbarth CA, Green J. Family of hemiplegic migraine and degeneration deafness and nystagmus. *Arch Neurol* 1970;23:201–209.
23. Delgado-Escueta AV, Greenberg DA, Treiman L. Mapping the gene for juvenile myoclonic epilepsy. *Epilepsia* 1989;30(Suppl 4):S8–S18.
24. Lehesjoki AE, Koskiniemi M, Sistonen P, et al. Localization of a gene for progressive myoclonus epilepsy to chromosome 21q22. *Proc Natl Acad Sci* 1991;88:3696–3699.
25. Miles DK, Holmes GL. Benign Neonatal Seizures. *J Clin Neurophysiol* 1990;7:369–379.
26. Leigh H, Lerner A. Transinhibitory seizures mimicking crescendo TIA's. *Neurology* 1990;40:165–166.
27. Tinuper P, Cerullo A, Cirignotta F, et al. Nocturnal paroxysmal dystonia with short lasting attacks: three cases with evidence of an epileptic frontal lobe origin of seizures. *Epilepsia* 1990;31:549–556.
28. Ozelius L, Kramer PL, Moskowitz CB, et al. Human gene for torsion dystonia located on chromosome 9q32–q34. *Neuron* 1989;2:1427–1434.
29. Tada H, Miyake S, Yamada M, Iwamoto H, Morooka K, Sakuragawa N. A patient with alternating hemiplegia in childhood. *No To Hattatsu* 1989;21:283–288.
30. Zupanc L, Dobkin JA, Perlman SB. Iodine 123 iodoamphetamine single photon emission computed tomography brain imaging in a child with alternating hemiplegia. *Ann Neurol* 1989;26:454–455.
31. Siemes H, Casaer P. Alternating hemiplegia in childhood. Clinical report and single photon emission computed tomography study. *Monatsschr Kinderheilkd* 1988;8:467–470.
32. Kanazawa O, Shirasaka Y, Hatori H, Okuno T, Mikawa H. Ictal ^{99m}Tc-HMPAO SPECT in alternating hemiplegia. *Pediatr Neurol* 1991;7:121–124.
33. Hattori H, Hashizuka S, Matsawko O, Murata R, Ueda T. Alternating hemiplegia in infants: a case report with abnormal findings in ABR (auditory brain stem response) and SPECT (single photon emission CT). *Jpn J Pediatr* 1989;42:77–82.
34. Nakamura Y, Nagano T, Mizuguchi M, Mizuno Y, Tamagawka K, Komiya K, Hirabayashi S. Alternating hemiplegia in infants: A case report. *No To Hattatsu* 1986;18:406–412.
35. Sakuragawa N, Arima M, Matsumoto S. Nationwide investigations of actual condition about alternating hemiplegia of infants. *Journal of the Japan Pediatric Society* 1988;92:892–898.
36. Sakuragwa N, Matsuo T, Kimura S, et al. Alternating hemiplegia in infancy: Two case reports and reduced regional blood flow in "CO$_2$ dynamic positron emission tomography." *Brain Dev* 1985; 7:207.
37. Dalla Bernardina B, Capovilla G, Trevisan E, et al. Alternating hemiplegia in childhood. In: Andermann F, Lugaresi E, eds. Migraine and epilepsy. Boston: Butterworths;1987:188–201.
38. Hosking G, Cavanagh N, Wilson J. Alternating hemiplegia: Complicated migraine of infancy. *Arch Dis Child* 1978;53:656–659.
39. Santanelli P, Guerrini R, Dravet C, Genton P, Bureau M, Farnarier G. Brainstem auditory evoked potentials in alternating hemiplegia: ictal vs interictal assessment of one case. *Clin Electroencephalogr* 1990;28:51–54.
40. Imai T, Minami R, Ishikawa Y, Okabe M, Matsumoto H. Reversible changes of somatosensory-evoked potentials in a child with alternating hemiplegia (Letter). *J Child Neurol* 1990;5:71–72.

41. Ishikawa Y, Imai T, Okabe M, et al. A case of alternating hemiplegia in infancy: ictal SSEP findings. *No To Hattatsu* 1989;21:495–497.
42. Schapira AVH. Mitochondrial disorders. *Curr Opin Neurol Neurosurg* 1990;3:425–530.
43. Campistol-Plana J, Sans-Fito A, Pineda-Marfa M, Fernandez-Alvarez E. Alternating hemiplegia in infancy: clinical features, clinical course and treatment based on three cases. *An Esp Pediatr* 1990; 32:336–338.
44. Salmon M, Wilson J. Drugs for alternating hemiplegia migraine (Letter). *Lancet* 1984;2:579.
45. Louis P. A double-blind placebo-controlled prophylactic study of flunarizine (Sibelium ®) in migraine. *Headache* 1981;21:235–239.

Alternating Hemiplegia of Childhood, edited by
Frederick Andermann, Jean Aicardi, and Federico Vigevano,
Raven Press, Ltd., New York © 1995.

17

Benign Familial Nocturnal Alternating Hemiplegia of Childhood

Eva Andermann, Frederick Andermann, *Kenneth Silver,
†Simon D. Levin, and Douglas L. Arnold

*Department of Neurology, Neurosurgery, and Pediatrics, McGill University, Montreal
Neurological Hospital and Institute, 3801 University Street, Montreal, Quebec H3A 2B4,
Canada; *Montreal Children's Hospital, Montreal, Quebec H3H 1P3, Canada; and
†Children's Hospital of Western Ontario, 800 Commissioners Road East,
London, Ontario N6C 2V5, Canada.*

In 1989 we studied a 2-year-old boy who had frequent attacks of alternating hemiplegia arising exclusively out of sleep. He would cry or moan, wake up, and then develop flaccid hemiplegia which recovered after he fell back to sleep. The attacks recurred several times a week. The child was neurologically normal. He was the only one of 10 children studied by our group to develop such episodes out of sleep but because of the typical appearance of the acute attacks he was included in the group presented in this volume. Over the years his development remained normal. Several months ago his mother reported that a brother born since the proband was last examined had developed an identical clinical picture.

On reviewing all available previously described cases with a view to genetic analysis, we noticed that Verret and Steele (1) in their original paper had described siblings who also had nocturnal onset alternating hemiplegia, and who eventually remitted. These children were not considered to have the disorder as defined by Aicardi and Krägeloh (2) and were therefore not included in their analysis. No follow-up was available. The siblings in the family we report here are considered to have a sleep-related and benign form of alternating hemiplegia of childhood (AHC). Recognition of this entity is particularly important from a prognostic point of view since it must be distinguished from the malignant, more common sporadic form of the disease.

PATIENT REPORTS

J.B. developed his first hemiplegic attack at 4½ months of age. He woke screaming 1½ hours after going to sleep and the parents noted that he was paralyzed on one side. Eventually he went back to sleep and when he woke in the morning he was well. Similar episodes then recurred, always during sleep and with increasing frequency.

He was born after a normal pregnancy, labor, and delivery at term. Apgar scores were 8 and 9. He had good birth weight but had some difficulty feeding shortly after birth and seemed to get tired after sucking for a few minutes. He received his first 3 DPT immunizations without complications.

Initially the attacks lasted about 5 minutes and occurred on an average of 3 times a week for a duration of minutes. Later they increased in length to about 20 minutes. Typically the child would go to sleep well. After approximately one or two hours he would cry, awaken, his eyes would open, and after a few seconds he would sit up, cry, mumble or whine, then start screaming, and become very irritable. A few seconds after arousal he had unilateral face, arm, and leg paralysis, or bilateral hemiplegia. If he was sitting he would slump onto the weak side at the onset of weakness. If the parents picked him up or stimulated him he could only move one side of the body. The face was weak and the arm was flaccid; the leg was less severely involved. In bilateral episodes the weakness was less severe but he would drool and had some difficulty breathing. He preferred to keep his eyes shut, was photophobic, and did not like to be disturbed. When the attacks had progressed he tried to talk but the words were garbled and incomprehensible. He seemed to understand what his parents were saying. Eventually he sighed, moaned, and fell asleep. When he awoke in the morning he was perfectly well. Attacks occurred only during night-time sleep and rarely during naps during the day. The mother noted that when he had a busy, exciting, or stimulating day he would be more likely to have an attack during sleep.

A CT scan, four-vessel arteriogram, and a PET scan were normal. An EEG showed focal slowing contralateral to the paralyzed side during an attack. Dystonic posturing and ocular movement abnormalities were not present during the episodes. Developmental milestones were normal. At 3½ years of age he was reinvestigated. During an attack with left-sided weakness the arm was flaccid, the leg was weak with increased reflexes, and he had a Babinski response on that side. Three polysomnograms showed delayed onset of REM sleep, and increased stages 3 and 4. A hemiplegic attack occurred during stage 4 sleep. No epileptic discharge was seen.

Initially he was treated with Dilantin which led to an increase in number and duration of attacks. Pizotyline and propranolol had no effect. Flunarizine 5 mg and later 7.5 mg at bedtime induced some improvement in the duration but not in the frequency of the episodes: average duration of attacks was reduced from 20 minutes to about 5 minutes. The density of the hemiplegia remained unchanged. Slurred or garbled speech was noted with attacks involving either side. Bilateral attacks were infrequent and in these the weakness was less severe. Their duration was similar to that of the unilateral ones. The neurological examination remained normal. The addition of 5 mg of clobazam reduced the frequency of episodes from three per week to one every week or week and a half. Attacks were reported to increase in frequency in relation to stress and sleep deprivation.

At the age of 5 his intelligence and neurological examination were again normal. He was now able to describe what he felt during his attacks. He stated that he had a pain in the chest and in the neck. When the attacks involved one side he could talk but he could not do so when they were on the other side. This implies an aphasic disturbance but the lateralization of speech disturbance could not be clarified further at that time.

M.B., the third son of this couple developed attacks of alternating hemiplegia arising out of sleep at the age of 4 months. He would wake 1–2 hours after falling asleep screaming and crying. The mother commented that his crying had the same tone and fury as that of his brother at the beginning of attacks. After a few seconds he became paralyzed on one side for about 10 minutes and then fell asleep again. When he awoke he was well. Attacks involved one side or the other but were never bilateral, unlike some of those of his brother.

The episodes were clustered; he could be 2 or 3 weeks without an occurrence and than have an attack 2 or 3 nights in a row.

Pregnancy, labor, and delivery were normal. His neurological examination and development were entirely normal at the age of 14 months.

Both brothers were studied at ages 5 years and 14 months, respectively. Investigations included HMPAO SPECT scans and EEGs outside of attacks and these were normal. Plasma amino acid profile, T4, TSH, lactic acid, pyruvate, somatosensory and brainstem auditory evoked responses, MRI scans, and chromosome studies in both were normal.

MAGNETIC RESONANCE SPECTROSCOPY

Abnormalities were found by magnetic resonance spectroscopy of muscle in patient J.B. at the age of 2 years. When spectroscopy was repeated at age 5 at a time when the duration of his attacks was much diminished in response to flunarizine and clobazam, the spectroscopic findings had returned to normal. MRS of muscle in the second affected boy (M.B.), in the unaffected brother, and in their parents was normal.

THE B. FAMILY

The father of the boys had episodes of tunnel vision as a child and episodes of severe common migraine with nausea and photophobia in adulthood. His nephew had epilepsy, probably generalized, but no migraine. The mother had only occasional recurrent headaches. A paternal aunt has severe migraine as does her son. A maternal aunt had migraine with visual aura but without hemiplegia.

The third child of the couple was normal. He was calm and phlegmatic, unlike his two active and high strung affected brothers.

DISCUSSION

The history and the findings during attacks in the proband led to a diagnosis of AHC. The unusual timing of the attacks arising out of sleep was not considered sufficient to discard this diagnosis although sleep-related attacks were not described in other patients with this disorder. On the other hand, cessation of attacks with sleep is classical in children with alternating hemiplegia and was present in this family as well. The actual sleep pattern recorded in polysomnograms showed no significant abnormality.

When the third child was found to be affected it became clear that this disorder is distinct from AHC. The mental and motor development of the affected boys has been normal and has remained so. The repeated episodes of hemiplegia and of speech or language disorder coupled with abnormal pyramidal neurological signs during attacks have not led to recognizable permanent deficit.

The familial nature of this affection is unlike the sporadic occurrence of the classical form. In that disorder only a pair of identical twins have been found to be affected. The siblings mentioned by Verret and Steele most likely had the disorder we describe here but unfortunately follow-up and the original records have not been available. Eventually however those siblings ceased having attacks and their development was described at the time as normal.

The relationship of this disorder to migraine is as intriguing as it is in the families of children with the sporadic or classical form. A history of classical and of common migraine is present in the families of both parents, and it is likely that the alternating hemiplegia in these children represents a migraine related disorder. Migraine is an extremely common disorder with a very wide range of diagnostic criteria. There is extreme variability in the requirements for a diagnosis depending on the neurologist's views, bias, conceptualization, and personal experience. This probably accounts for the variance in accepting a relationship of classical or typical alternating hemiplegia to migraine.

The laboratory investigations carried out in this family have shown no consistent abnormalities. In this they tend to resemble other children with alternating hemiplegia. Magnetic resonance spectroscopy has shown no abnormality in the younger child and the abnormalities in the older boy were no longer present as he matured. Serial MR spectroscopic investigations over time, including studies during and between attacks, and during periods of greater or lesser activity should lead to further clarification.

More prolonged follow-up is required to confirm the benign nature of this syndrome. Once it is recognized as a separate entity it is quite likely that additional patients will be diagnosed. As children mature they should be able to provide additional details which could lead to further clarification.

Several forms of alternating hemiplegia with onset in childhood are now recognized in addition to the classical disorder: the dominant disease described by Mikati (see Chapter 16) paroxysmal symptomatic alternating dystonia with hemiparesis (in a patient with basal ganglia disease, probably Hallervorden-Spatz (see Chapter 19), and migraine coma, an unusual condition with hemiplegic migraine as a cardinal manifestation (see Chapter 22). The tendency to both alternating and at times bilateral attacks seems to be common to all these conditions and suggests a vascular factor or etiology in all. Abnormalities of energy metabolism however may also play an important role in the various forms of alternating hemiplegia and are increasingly studied in these disorders.

REFERENCES

1. Verret S, Steele JC. Alternating hemiplegia in childhood: a report of eight patients with complicated migraine beginning in infancy. *Pediatrics* 1971;47:675–680.
2. Krägeloh I, Aicardi J. Alternating hemiplegia in infants: report of five cases. *Dev Med Child Neurol* 1980;22:784–791.

Alternating Hemiplegia of Childhood, edited by
Frederick Andermann, Jean Aicardi, and Federico Vigevano,
Raven Press, Ltd., New York © 1995.

18

Infantile Hypotonia and Paroxysmal Dystonia

A Variant of Alternating Hemiplegia of Childhood

Frederick Andermann, *Shunsuke Ohtahara, Eva Andermann,
†Peter R. Camfield, and *Katsuhiro Kobayashi

*Department of Neurology and Neurosurgery, McGill University,
Montreal Neurological Hospital and Institute, 3801 University Street,
Montreal, Quebec H3A 2B4, Canada; *Department of Child Neurology,
Okayama University Medical School, 5-1, Shikatacho-2 chome,
Okayama 700, Japan; and †Department of Pediatrics, Dalhousie University,
Halifax, Nova Scotia B3J 3G9, Canada.*

Alternating hemiplegia of childhood (AHC) first described by Verret and Steele in 1971 (1) was more fully characterized by Jean Aicardi almost 10 years later (2,3). At the international symposium on this disorder held in Rome in January 1992 the relatively homogenous clinical picture was again stressed (see Chapters 1 and 2). The disorder becomes apparent from birth or early life with persistent hypotonia and episodic dystonic posturing occurring early, followed by hemiplegic attacks which occur either alone or in association with the dystonic events. The episodes of hemiplegia involve alternate sides and may last for minutes but usually for hours or days. The dystonic episodes become progressively less apparent but the hemiplegic attacks persist. Later in childhood or adolescence a permanent movement disorder, choreoathetotic, choreic, or dystonic becomes apparent. The disease seems progressive particularly in the early stages. The children are, or become, usually mildly to severely retarded. A relationship of this disorder to migraine has been postulated early (4). Treatment with flunarizine, a calcium channel blocker, usually reduces the intensity, but more rarely the frequency of the attacks (5–7).

At the International Symposium on Alternating Hemiplegia of Childhood, two patients with hypotonia and episodic paroxysmal dystonia who did not develop early hemiplegic attacks were discussed. Because of some characteristic clinical features their disorder may be considered to represent a variant of AHC. Further evidence for this view is provided by the eventual development of alternating hemiplegia in the second decade of life in one of these children and by her response to flunarizine.

The purpose of this chapter is to describe this paroxysmal movement disorder of childhood which should be considered in the differential diagnosis of paroxysmal dystonic events.

PATIENT REPORTS

Patient 1 (M.T.), a 3½-year-old Acadian girl was the only child of nonconsanguineous parents, born by breech delivery without evidence of anoxia. She was considered to be normal until the age of 4 months when she developed episodes of both eyes turning up and to the left with only minimal rotation of the head. She was hypotonic at the time. Several months later the attacks changed: she developed dystonia with turning of both head and eyes to the left and extension of the left arm and leg. These episodes lasted from minutes to hours and occurred several times a week. She was conscious during the attacks which could be precipitated by excitement and ceased after falling asleep even for a few minutes. She has had no monocular nystagmus or hemiplegia with her attacks and no epileptic seizures. The mother had common migraine.

At age 3½ years attacks occurred virtually every day with possibly 2 or 3 days a month without an attack. They varied in their timing during the day and lasted from 10 minutes to 30 minutes. She remained responsive to people around her by continuing to smile with stimulation. She was strikingly hypotonic and had little head control. Her eye movements were full, her smile was abundant and symmetric. She could not stand alone. She did not maintain herself independently sitting but could take some weight on her legs while held standing. Her deep tendon reflexes were brisk. She spoke a few words and was moderately retarded mentally. She could identify about 30 different objects on a picture board. She used her index finger pointing. She did not seem to use the picture board for communication spontaneously, rather she just pointed on command to the various pictures.

EEGs, MRI, and MRS were normal. The attacks did not respond to phenytoin, carbamazepine, clobazam, and flunarizine.

Patient 2, (S.I), a 17-year-old Japanese girl was delivered with mild asphyxia after a 40-week normal pregnancy. Birth weight was 3,520 g.

She attained head control at 5 months of age. During a febrile illness at 7 months of age, she had a dystonic episode with upward deviation of the eyes which lasted for 2 days. Similar spontaneous episodes lasting 10 minutes to several hours then recurred several times a month. Consciousness was not disturbed during the attacks.

She began to say words at 12 months, walked at 15 months, and spoke in sentences at 1½ years of age.

At the age of 2 years she developed opisthotonus during the dystonic events. There was still no impairment of consciousness or hemiplegia with these episodes.

At age 12 years, the episodes changed: she had stiffening of the right extremities lasting 10 minutes to 2 hours without impairment of consciousness. Attacks occurred only while awake, 2 to 16 times per month, and were not induced by movement.

At 14 years she was clumsy, had choreoathetosis of the upper extremities, and bilateral hyperreflexia. Her IQ was 86 on the Wechsler Intelligence Scale for Children (WISC). The attacks consisted of stiffening and dystonia of right extremities and hyperextension of the trunk. At times she would also have flaccid hemiplegia during the episodes. Ankle clonus was observed on the hemiplegic side during the attacks, but not in between. She had no Babinski response or autonomic signs. Similar but left-sided attacks now occurred independently, several times a week as well.

The EEG showed mildly dysrhythmic background activity (Fig. 1). EEG topographic mapping, using significance probability mapping (8), showed an increase of equivalent potentials, or square root values of power, compared with age-matched normative data (9) in the theta band (4.0–8.0 Hz) over both frontal region, though there was no abnormal theta activity in the visually interpreted EEG. There was no difference between ictal and interictal periods. (Fig. 2) Delta band (2.0–4.0 Hz) equivalent potentials were within normal limits. Cerebral blood flow measured between attacks by Xenon-enhanced computed tomography and ^{123}I-iodoamphetamine SPECT showed slight hypoperfusion of both thalami (Fig. 3). Laboratory investigations are summarized in Table 1 (10–14). At the age of 15 years flunarizine was prescribed. After the 35th day attacks ceased. Six months later she began to take the medication irregularly and some attacks returned. They ceased again when the medication was reintroduced.

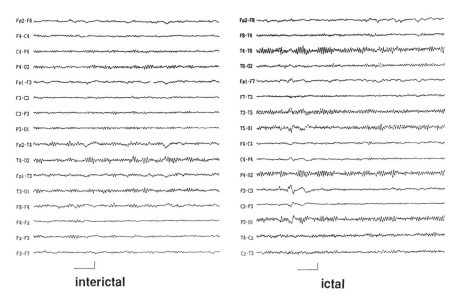

interictal   ictal

FIG. 1. Awake EEG of patient 2 at 14½ years of age during interictal (*Left*) and ictal (*Right*) periods. Calibrations: 1 sec and 100 μV.

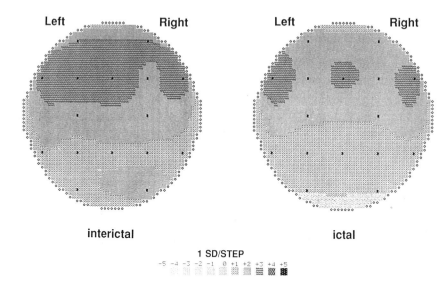

interictal   ictal

1 SD/STEP

−5 −4 −3 −2 −1 0 +1 +2 +3 +4 +5

FIG. 2. Theta band (4–8 Hz) EEG topograms of patient 2 at 14½ years of age using significance probability mapping. Increase of the equivalent potentials is shown in both frontal regions compared with age-matched normative data. There was no evident difference between interictal (*Left*) and ictal (*Right*) periods.

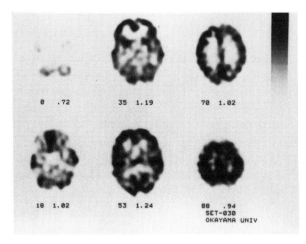

FIG. 3. Interictal ^{123}I-iodoamphetamine SPECT scan of patient 2 at 14½ years of age showing a tendency to hypoperfusion in both thalami.

TABLE 1. *Laboratory examinations of patient 2*

Electrolytes: Between attacks; Na 141 mmol/l, K 4.0 mmol/l, Cl 105 mmol/l, Ca 8.9 mg/dl, inorganic phosphate (IP) 4.5 mg/dl, Mg 2.1 mg/dl. During an attack; Na 138 mmol/l, K 4.0 mmol/l, Cl 106 mmol/l, Ca 8.5 mg/dl, IP 4.2 mg/dl, Mg 1.7 mg/dl.

Hematology: Erythrocyte count $4.44 \times 10^6/\mu$l, hemoglobin 12.5g/dl, hematocrit 37.2%, platelet count $265 \times 10^3/\mu$l, leukocyte count $5.4 \times 10^3/\mu$l (normal differential cell counts).
Bleeding time: 3 minutes 30 seconds.
Coagulation study: Prothrombin time 13.4 sec, activated partial thromboplastin time 38.9 sec, fibrinogen 286 mg/dl.

Blood-lactate: 10 mg/dl, pyruvate 0.9 mg/dl.

Cerebrospinal fluid: Initial pressure 70 mmH$_2$O, cells 0/ml, total protein 20 mg/dl, glucose 45 mg/dl.

Ceruloplasmin: 24.2 mg/dl.

Cryoglobulins: Negative.

Cranial computed tomography and magnetic resonance imaging: normal.

Evoked potential studies (auditory brainstem responses, visual evoked potentials, and photoevoked eyelid microvibration): Normal between and during attacks compared with age-matched normative data (10–12).

Carotid and vertebral angiography: No abnormality.

Cerebral blood flow measurement by transcranial Doppler ultrasound in the middle cerebral and basilar arteries: Normal both during ictal and interictal period compared with age-matched normative data (13–14).

DISCUSSION

These two children developed paroxysmal dystonic attacks early in life. In addition, the first child was strikingly hypotonic and had considerable delay in motor development. Mental functions were difficult to assess accurately but she appeared severely retarded. At age 3½ years she has had no episodic hemiplegia with the dystonic attacks.

The second patient also had early generalized dystonic attacks and these became lateralized around the age of 12. At 14 it became clear that she had flaccid hemiparesis in association with the attacks and that these involved both sides independently. She had choreoathetosis but her intelligence was relatively normal.

Long-term follow-up should also clarify the problem of the first patient since the second child developed her hemiplegic attacks only in the second decade of life.

Many of the clinical features of the children, particularly, family history of migraine, hypotonia, and triggering of attacks by excitement and their cessation with even short naps are characteristic of AHC. The hemiplegic attacks are a cardinal feature of that condition and occur invariably before 18 months of age; patients with the other features of this condition but without the hemiplegia have not been described so far. Yet it is likely that the two children presented here suffer from an atypical form of this disorder.

AHC usually responds to a degree to the administration of flunarizine, a calcium channel blocker (5–7): Occasionally attacks cease completely in response to this medication as in the second patient but some do not respond, as the first child. The attacks of these patients do not represent epileptic seizures and none of the known paroxysmal movement disorders of childhood are suggested by the clinical picture. In the differential diagnosis, pyruvate dehydrogenase deficiency, Leigh's disease, the classical forms of hemiplegic migraine, and MELAS syndrome must be considered.

There is much debate about the cause of AHC: a relationship to migraine has been postulated (4,7) but this is not universally accepted (3). The first child's mother clearly had common migraine; in view of the invariable occurrence of migraine in one or both parents in our experience with 10 patients (7) this association appears significant. The second author found no such family history in the second patient. This may represent a difference in the diagnostic criteria for migraine between the two centers.

Patients with alternating hemiplegia usually have MRS abnormalities suggesting mitochondrial dysfunction (see Chapter 15) but the specific significance of these abnormalities remains unclear. The second patient had normal serum lactate and pyruvate but such normal determinations are not exceptional in patients with other forms of proven mitochondrial disease.

This variant of alternating hemiplegia should be considered in the investigation of infants with paroxysmal dystonic phenomena. Its mechanism will be better understood when the pathogenesis of the typical form of AHC is clarified

CONCLUSION

Two children had early onset of hypotonia and frequent episodes of paroxysmal dystonia. The dystonic episodes were abolished by even brief naps. One child had a clear family history of migraine but this was not elicited in the second child. One of the children developed alternating hemiplegia in the second decade; the other has had no hemiplegic episodes by age 3½ years. In the classical form episodes of alternating hemiplegia invariably develop before the age of 18 months. These children seem to have a variant of the now well recognized picture of AHC but other etiologies, as yet undetermined must be considered as well. This variant must be considered in the differential diagnosis of paroxysmal dystonia in childhood.

REFERENCES

1. Verret S, Steele JC. Alternating hemiplegia in childhood; A report of eight patients with complicated migraine beginning in infancy. *Pediatrics* 1971;47:675–680.
2. Krägeloh I, Aicardi J. Alternating hemiplegia in infants: Report of five cases. *Dev Med Child Neurol* 1980;22:784–791.
3. Aicardi J. Alternating hemiplegia of childhood. *Int Pediatr* 1987:2;115–119.

4. Hosking GP, Cavanagh NPC, Wilson J. Alternating hemiplegia: complicated migraine of infancy. *Arch Dis Child* 1978;53:656–659.
5. Casaer P, Azou M. Flunarizine in alternating hemiplegia in childhood. *Lancet* 1984;2:579.
6. Casaer P. Flunarizine in alternating hemiplegia in childhood. An international study in 12 children. *Neuropediatrics* 1987;18:191–195.
7. Silver R, Andermann F. Alternating hemiplegia of childhood: A study of 10 patients and results of flunarizine treatment, *Neurology* 1993;43(1):36–41.
8. Duffy FH, Bartels PH, Burchfiel JL. Significance probability mapping: An aid in the topographic analysis of brain electrical activity. *Electroencephalogr Clin Neurophysiol* 1981;51:455–462.
9. Yoshida H. Development of EEG during infancy and childhood by EEG topographic mapping. *Jpn J Electroencephalogr Electromyogr* 1984;12:248–260.
10. Iyoda K. Development of auditory brainstem response during infancy and childhood. *Jpn J Electroencephalogr Electromyogr* 1992;20:44–52.
11. Miyake S, Terasaki T, Iyoda K, Yoshida H, Ohtahara S. A study on visual evoked potentials during infancy and childhood. *Jpn J Electroencephalogr Electromyogr* 1988;12:122–128.
12. Sanada S, Kobayashi K, Murakami N, Miyake S, Ohtahara S. Studies on photo-evoked eyelid microvibration. II. Developmental change. *Jpn J Electroencephalogr Electromyogr* 1987;15:36–41.
13. Horiuchi I. Developmental change and physiological variation of blood flow velocity of the basilar artery. *Okayama Igakkai Zasshi* 1991;103:19–29.
14. Murakami N. A study on intracranial hemodynamics by Doppler ultrasound. *No To Hattatsu* 1988;20:279–287.

Alternating Hemiplegia of Childhood, edited by
Frederick Andermann, Jean Aicardi, and Federico Vigevano,
Raven Press, Ltd., New York © 1995.

19

Symptomatic Alternating Paroxysmal Dystonia and Hemiplegia

Yvonne M. Hart, * Kevin Farrell, †Donatella Tampieri,
††Eva Andermann and ††Frederick Andermann

*Department of Neurology, Atkinson Morley's Hospital, Wimbledon, London SW20 ONE England; *Division of Neurology, Department of Pediatrics, University of British Columbia, Vancouver, British Columbia V6H 3V4 Canada; †Department of Radiology and ††Departments of Neurology, Neurosurgery, and Pediatrics, McGill University, Montreal Neurological Hospital and Institute, 3801 University Street, Montreal, Quebec, H3A 2B4 Canada*

Alternating hemiplegia of childhood (AHC) typically develops in children under the age of 18 months who are neurologically normal, or in some instances in children with hypotonia and psychomotor retardation. Other neurological deficits occur later in the disease (see Chapters 1, 2). We have examined one child with a long-standing neurological disorder causing motor delay, spasticity, and ataxia, who at the age of 10 years developed episodes of abnormal movements affecting either side of the body, or, more rarely, both sides simultaneously, similar in this respect to the episodes which occur in AHC. These attacks were initially thought to be epileptic, but with time it became clear that they represented paroxysmal dystonia, occurring in association with demonstrable progressive basal ganglia disease. Examination showed that she had weakness of the involved side during these episodes. The underlying neurological condition may represent an unusual form of Hallervorden-Spatz disease.

CLINICAL HISTORY

The patient was a 13-year-old girl born of nonconsanguineous Caucasian parents. There was no history of neurological disorder on the father's side, but a maternal uncle had a history of tremor, not associated with ataxia, intellectual deterioration, or other problems. The mother suffered from common migraine, and the patient's brother, aged 14, was being treated for an attention-deficit disorder.

Pregnancy and delivery were normal, and the patient weighed 7 lb 5 oz at birth. There were no perinatal problems. She was noted to be hypotonic in the first 2 months of life, and her motor milestones were delayed: she first sat independently at 9 months and walked at 22 months. She was said to have been "always clumsy." At the age of 2 she was noted to have tremor and ataxia which have progressed, initially slowly but at an accelerating pace from the age of 8. At the age of 12 years she started to use a walker. She also became increasingly dysarthric.

She first developed episodes of hemiparesis at the age of 10. These occurred during sleep, and she would be found on the floor by her parents who were wakened by her shouting. She had dystonic posturing of the right arm and leg, associated with pain and weakness. She also had right-sided facial weakness of the upper motor neuron type, and difficulty speaking because of increased dysarthria, but could answer simple questions and obey commands. The episodes ended abruptly after 15 to 30 minutes, when the patient would smile and say "It's over."

Treatment with carbamazepine was instituted and the episodes improved for 2 to 3 months, only to recur during waking as well as in sleep. They were not helped by acetazolamide or clobazam, nor by lorazepam, diazepam, or paraldehyde given acutely. Trials of levodopa and anticholinergic agents were similarly unhelpful.

The frequency and duration of the episodes increased over the years, and she could have 2 or 3 in a day, rarely being free of them for more than a few days. During the day, they occurred more frequently when she was active. They could last up to one hour. On a few occasions (approximately 5% of the total) the dystonic posturing and hemiparesis affected the left side of the body instead of the right. Following withdrawal of carbamazepine during assessment in hospital she developed attacks involving both sides simultaneously, during which she was mute and experienced drooling, difficulty with breathing, and considerable distress.

On examination her head circumference, height, and weight were at the fifth percentile. Cardiovascular, respiratory, and abdominal examination was normal, and she had no skeletal deformities or skin lesions. She had hypermetric saccades but full external ocular movements, and normal visual fields, acuity and fundi. She had a cerebellar dysarthria and a tendency to drool. Examination of the cranial nerves was otherwise normal. She had marked spasticity of all four limbs, with hyperactive reflexes and ankle clonus bilaterally, but normal power except during her attacks. She had bilateral extensor plantar responses, head titubation, intention tremor, and a very ataxic gait. Sensory examination was normal.

Repeated neuropsychological testing did not show any definite evidence of intellectual deterioration. However, she complained of difficulty in moving her eyes and had largely stopped reading. Her dysarthria and ataxia also impeded her work. She used a computer and had special help at school, where she attended grade 7 in a modified program.

Blood tests, including lactate, ammonia, thyroid function, cholesterol, triglycerides, ceruloplasmin, copper, alpha-fetoprotein, renal function, calcium, and magnesium were normal. Arylsulfatase A, hexosaminidase, plasma very long chain fatty acids, and urinary oligosaccharides were also normal. There was no abnormality of plasma and cerebrospinal fluid (CSF) amino acids, which were tested on several occasions. CSF protein was normal, without oligoclonal bands: measles and rubella antibodies were not detected. CSF lactate was normal.

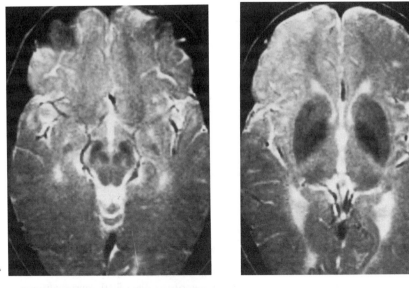

A

B

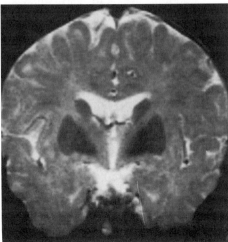

C

FIG. 1. A–C. Axial **(A, B)** and coronal **(C)** T_2 weighted images demonstrating the hypointense signals in the red nuclei, substantia nigra, basal ganglia, and thalamic pulvinar. The hyperintensities involving the U-fibers are better displayed on the coronal view.

CT scan performed on four occasions showed no abnormality. However, MRI scan of the head showed marked reduction in signal intensity from the basal ganglia, particularly in the globus pallidus, but also in the putamen, red nucleus, substantia nigra, the caudate nucleus and thalamic pulvinar on both sides. In addition some white matter signal changes were present in the region of the U fibers (Fig. 1).

EKG was normal, as were nerve conduction studies in the upper and lower limbs. EEG showed a mildly dysrhythmic background, with intermittent delta activity over the frontal regions bilaterally. EEG during the attacks was contaminated with movement artifact rendering interpretation difficult. Brainstem auditory evoked responses showed delayed V waves bilaterally. Visual evoked responses showed delayed responses to monocular pattern reversal stimuli on both sides.

Muscle biopsy performed at the age of 11 showed no ragged red fibers. Mitochondrial and muscle enzyme studies were normal. Skin fibroblast culture showed normal pyruvate dehydrogenase activity.

DISCUSSION

This girl presented with a progressive neurological disease involving the extra-pyramidal, pyramidal, and cerebellar systems. She had documented motor delay and some ataxia before the age of 8, but there was relatively little if any progression till then. Subsequent steady deterioration and frequent episodes of paroxysmal dystonia developed.

The similarity in the temporal patterns between the episodes of dystonia and hemiparesis occurring in this patient with the episodes of paralysis seen in AHC is striking. The duration of attacks, their great frequency, and above all the alternating side or bilateral involvement are very similar, and dystonic features are well recognized during the hemiplegic episodes, particularly early in the course of the illness (1). The family history of migraine is also the rule in families of children with alternating hemiplegia. However, there are some important differences. First, although our patient had some neurological symptoms at an early age, the onset of the episodes of dystonia and hemiparesis was not until the age of 10 years, while episodes of hemiplegia in AHC present before the age of 18 months (2). Second, while some patients with this syndrome have had prior psychomotor retardation (3), and though Verret and Steele (4) described one patient as having always shown "mild spasticity of the legs, incoordination of the extremities, choreoathetosis of the hands, and dystonic posturing of the arms," pre-existing progressive neurological abnormalities of the type described in our patient are not a feature. The neurological problems which she has subsequently developed are similarly unlike those usually described, which include mental retardation, choreoathetosis, sometimes seizures, and rarely hemiparesis (1–4). Finally, the MRI scan of patients with AHC does not show abnormalities other than slight atrophy, even when fixed deficits are present.

Episodes of paroxysmal unilateral (or sometimes bilateral) dystonic posturing have long been recognized both in association with other neurological symptoms and independently, often on a familial basis. Sterling (5) reported spasms, lasting up to several hours and involving one or more limbs and sometimes the face, in patients who have had encephalitis lethargica. Matthews (6) and Joynt and Green (7) reported tonic spasms occurring in association with multiple sclerosis, but these invariably lasted at most only a few minutes. Familial paroxysmal choreoathetosis, with episodes lasting from a few minutes to 2 hours, was described by Mount and Reback in 1940 (8) in a patient with no other neurological symptoms (and normal neurological examination except for questionable glove and stocking sensory loss): other reports were provided by Forssman in 1961 and Lance in 1963 (9,10). The dystonic component of many of these episodes was recognized by Richards and Barnett (11), who introduced the term *paroxysmal dystonic choreoathetosis*, and Lance (12) reported episodes of choreoathetosis in one member of a family, while two other members had dystonic spasms, with mild choreoathetoid movements. The duration of these episodes varied from seconds to a few hours, and they were somewhat similar to the attacks seen in our patient, although in neither the familial nor sporadic forms has hemiparesis been stressed. It is of interest, however, that an autosomal dominant form of AHC has recently been described (see Chapter 16). Kertesz (13) further defined the syndrome of paroxysmal kinesigenic choreoathetosis in which episodes of dystonia are induced by movement, and which is often inherited in an autosomal dominant manner, though sporadic cases also occur. In the latter syndrome the episodes usually respond to antiepileptic medication, and are generally short-lived, lasting seconds or minutes, unlike our patient's attacks.

There are numerous causes of secondary dystonia occurring in childhood, though the extent to which the dystonia is paroxysmal varies. They include Leigh's disease, neuronal ceroid lipofuscinosis, ataxia telangiectasia, pyruvate dehydrogenase deficiency, GM_1 gangliosidosis, homocystinuria, glutaric acidemia, metachromatic leukodystrophy, Pelizaeus-Merzbacher disease, and Wilson's disease (14), all of which can be excluded in our patient on the basis of the clinical features or laboratory findings. Burke et al. (15) reported the occurrence of dystonia delayed for 1 to 14 years after a nonprogressive cerebral insult. Dystonia with diurnal variation (16) was also considered in our patient, but there was no diurnal variation in her dystonia nor any response to levodopa therapy to suggest this diagnosis.

Hallervorden-Spatz disease, an autosomal recessive disorder, was suggested by the MRI scan appearance. The imaging features described in Hallervorden-Spatz disease include a marked exaggeration of the low signal normally seen on T_2-weighted images in the globus pallidus (17–20). The low signal area often surrounds an area of high signal, the so-called "eye-of-the-tiger" sign, but the extent to which this is a constant feature is uncertain: while it was described in all the cases reported by Savoiardo et al. (21), it has only been stressed in a few other reports. White matter changes have been described in a periependymal distribution in patients with atypical clinical presentations (22). Dooling et al. (23) distinguished two types of Hallervorden-Spatz disease according to whether pathological involvement of the pars reticulata of the substantia nigra was present in addition to the involvement of the globus pallidus. These authors also delineated a third group of patients with typical pallidonigral changes pathologically, but atypical clinical histories. They felt that it was not reasonable to include such patients in the group with Hallervorden-Spatz disease, and similar MRI abnormalities in other diseases have been described (24–26). None of Dooling's latter group had symptoms resembling those of our patient. The CT scan in Hallervorden-Spatz disease may be normal, as in our patient, or show areas of calcification in the medial part of the pallidum (21). The diagnosis of this disease, however, cannot be definitely confirmed in life, and the paroxysmal nature of our patient's dystonia and hemiparesis has not been described in this condition. Clinically, although spasticity is well recognized in Hallervorden-Spatz disease, cerebellar signs are not prominent.

Our patient thus presents an unusual picture of a progressive neurological disease including pyramidal, extrapyramidal, and cerebellar features, with radiological features reminiscent of Hallervorden-Spatz disease, in association with symptomatic alternating paroxysmal dystonia and hemiparesis.

REFERENCES

1. Dalla Bernardina B, Capovilla G, Trevisan E, Colamaria V, Andrighetto G, Fontana E, Tassinari CA. Alternating hemiplegia in childhood. In: Andermann F, Lugaresi E, eds. Migraine and epilepsy. Boston: Butterworths; 1987;189–201.
2. Krägeloh I, Aicardi J. Alternating hemiplegia in infants: Report of five cases. *Dev Med Child Neurol* 1980;22:784–791.
3. Dittrich J, Havlová M, Nevšimalová S. Paroxysmal hemipareses in childhood. *Dev Med Child Neurol* 1979;21:800–807.
4. Verret S, Steele JC. Alternating hemiplegia in childhood: A report of eight patients with complicated migraine beginning in infancy. *Pediatrics* 1971;47:675–680.
5. Sterling W. Le type spasmodique tétanoide et tétaniforme de l'encéphalite épidémique: remarques sur l'épilepsie "extra-pyramidale." *Rev Neurol* (Paris) 1924;31:484–492.
6. Matthews WB. Tonic seizures in disseminated sclerosis. *Brain* 1958;81:193–206.
7. Joynt RJ, Green D. Tonic seizures as a manifestation of multiple sclerosis. *Arch Neurol* 1962;6: 293–299.
8. Mount LA, Reback S. Familial paroxysmal choreoathetosis: preliminary report on a hitherto undescribed clinical syndrome. *Arch Neurol Psychiatr* 1940;44:841–847.
9. Forssman H. Heteditary disorder characterized by attacks of muscular contractions, induced by alcohol amongst other factors. *Acta Med Scand* 1961;170,517–533.
10. Lance JW. Sporadic and familial varieties of tonic seizures. *J Neurol Neurosurg Psychiatr* 1963;26: 51–59.
11. Richards RN, Barnett HJM. Paroxysmal dystonic choreoathetosis: A family study and review of the literature. *Neurology* 1968;18:461–469.
12. Lance JW. Familial paroxysmal dystonic choreoathetosis and its differentiation from related syndromes. *Ann Neurol* 1977;2:285–293.
13. Kertesz A. Paroxysmal kinesigenic choreoathetosis: an entity within the paroxysmal choreoathetosis syndrome: description of 10 cases, including 1 autopsied. *Neurology* 1967;17:680–690.
14. Calne DB, Lang AE. Secondary dystonia. *Adv Neurol* 1988;50:9–33.
15. Burke RE, Fahn S, Gold AP. Delayed onset dystonia in patients with 'static' encephalopathy. *J Neurol Neurosurg Psychiatr* 1980;44:460.
16. Segawa M, Nomura Y, Kase M. Hereditary progressive dystonia with marked diurnal fluctuation: clinicopathophysiological identification in reference to juvenile Parkinson's disease. *Adv Neurol* 1987;45:227.
17. Tanfani G, Mascalchi M, Dal Pozzo GC, Taverni N, Saia A, Trevisan C. MR imaging in a case of Hallervorden-Spatz disease. *J Comput Assist Tomogr* 1987;11:1057–1058.
18. Sethi KD, Adams RJ, Loring DW, El Gammal T. Hallervorden-Spatz syndrome: clinical and magnetic resonance imaging correlations. *Ann Neurol* 1988;24:692–694.
19. Mutoh K, Okuno T, Ito M, Nakano S, Mikawa H, Fujisawa I, Asato R. MR imaging of a group I case of Hallervorden-Spatz disease. *J Comput Assist Tomogr* 1988;12:851–853.
20. Schaffert DA, Johnsen SD, Johnson PC, Drayer BP. Magnetic resonance imaging in pathologically proven Hallervorden-Spatz disease. *Neurology* 1989;39;440–442.
21. Savoiardo M, Halliday WC, Nardocci N, Strada L, D'Incerti L, Angelini L, Rumi V, Tesoro-Tess JD. Hallervorden-Spatz disease: MR and pathologic findings. *AJNR* 1993;14:155–162.
22. Littrup PJ, Gebarski SS. MR imaging of Hallervorden-Spatz disease. *J Comput Assist Tomogr* 1985;9:491–493.
23. Dooling EC, Schoene WC, Richardson EP. Hallervorden-Spatz syndrome. *Arch Neurol* 1974;30: 70–83.
24. Drayer BP, Olanow W, Burger P, Johnson JT, Herfkens R, Riederer S. Parkinson plus syndrome: diagnosis using high field MR imaging of brain iron. *Radiology* 1986;159:493–498.
25. Drayer B, Burger P, Hurwitz B, Dawson D, Cain J. Reduced signal intensity on MR images of thalamus and putamen in multiple sclerosis: increased iron content? *AJNR* 1987;8:413–419.
26. Pastakia B, Polinsky R, Di Chiro G, Simmons JT, Brown R, Wener L. Multiple system atrophy (Shy-Drager syndrome): MR imaging. *Radiology* 1986;159:499–502.

Alternating Hemiplegia of Childhood, edited by
Frederick Andermann, Jean Aicardi, and Federico Vigevano,
Raven Press, Ltd., New York © 1995.

20

Alternating Hemiplegia of Childhood Associated with Mitochondrial Disease

A Deficiency of Pyruvate Dehydrogenase

*Kenneth Silver, *Charles Scriver, †Douglas L. Arnold,
§Brian Robinson, and †Frederick Andermann

*Departments of Neurology, Neurosurgery, and Pediatrics, McGill University; †Montreal
Neurological Hospital and Institute, 3801 University Street, Quebec H3A 2B4, Canada;
*Montreal Children's Hospital, Montreal, Quebec H3H 1P3, Canada; and §Department of
Pathology, The Hospital for Sick Children, Toronto, Ontario M5G 1X8, Canada.*

The etiology and pathophysiological mechanisms of alternating hemiplegia of child-hood (AHC) are unknown. The differential diagnosis includes vascular disorders, epilepsy, paroxysmal movement disorders and metabolic disease (1). A recent study using magnetic resonance spectroscopy (MRS) demonstrated evidence for mito-chondrial dysfunction in patients with AHC (2; see Chapter 15).

Neurological diseases associated with mitochondrial dysfunction have increas-ingly been recognized over the past decade. The clinical manifestations of these patients are extremely varied (3). The most frequent disorders of mitochondrial function are due to defects of the pyruvate dehydrogenase complex(PDHC). The PDHC macromolecule assembly of proteins carries out oxidative decarboxylation of pyruvate which is the product of glycolysis. Cytosolic pyruvate is transported across the mitochondrial membrane where in the matrix, it is decarboxylated and activated to acetyl CoA by PDHC. Defects of the PDHC characteristically result in elevated levels of pyruvate, lactate, and alanine. The clinical manifestations of patients with PDHC deficiency can vary from neonatal death to benign intermittent ataxia (4). We present a patient with PDHC deficiency and episodes of alternating hemiplegia and compare him to other patients with the syndrome of AHC.

PATIENT REPORT

A 5-year-old boy was born after a normal term pregnancy and delivery to healthy nonconsanguineous parents. The one, five, and ten minute Apgar scores were 9, 10, and 10, respectively, and there were no perinatal difficulties. Birth weight was 3.32 kg, length 50 cm, and head circumference 35 cm; all at the 50th percentile. There were no family members with migraine, seizures, developmental, or neurological disorders. Since birth he had frequent regurgitation which improved after 10 months. An upper GI study confirmed gastroesophageal reflux. At 8 months of age he was noted to have developmental delay with head lag and was unable to sit or grasp objects. However, by 15 months of age he was able to accomplish these milestones and to say a few words. At 3 years of age he could walk and developed a pincer grasp. At 5 years he talked in two word phrases with a vocabulary of 30 words. Over the years his height, weight, and head circumference has fallen below the fifth percentile(Fig. 1).

At 1½ years of age he started to have episodes of unilateral weakness. The attacks occurred about once per month and involved the arm, face, and leg. During these he was unable to lift his arm or grasp objects. When he tried to walk his leg gave way and he would fall. The hemiplegia lasted for at least one hour. After he went to sleep he would waken hours later without any evidence of the hemiparesis. Prior to the attacks there was no aura, color change of the extremities, change in respiratory pattern, nor were abnormal movements such as dystonia, choreoathetosis, nystagmus, or ocular motor abnormalities present. Most of the attacks occurred spontaneously but on occasion they were provoked by upper respiratory infections or gastroenteritis. On such occasions he could have up to four attacks in one month. Two episodes of weakness were generalized and not associated with loss of consciousness. He has not had any seizures nor ataxia with the attacks and they equally involved either side of the body.

At 5 years of age he was an alert, hyperactive, distractible boy who spoke few words and could follow simple commands. Head circumference was just below the second percentile. There was no nystagmus and he had full extra-ocular movements. The fundi, cranial nerves, motor examination, and stretch responses were normal. He had a bilateral Babinski response and decreased rapid alternating movements. His gait was mildly wide based but not ataxic. He did not have any movement disorder, organomegaly, or dysmorphic features.

Investigations revealed a compensated metabolic acidosis, pH 7.40, pCO_2 20 mmHg, bicarbonate 13 MEq/L, hydrogen ion concentration 40, base excess -9, with increased anion gap of 20.7. Urinalysis, serum glucose, electrolytes, total protein, bilirubin, AST, ALT, alkaline phosphatase, calcium, phosphorus, BUN, creatinine, T4, TSH, ammonia, free and total carnitine, CBC and differential were normal. IgG and IgM titers for CMV, rubella, toxoplasmosis, and VDRL were negative. Serum lactate was increased to 6.7 mmol/L (normal 0.6–2.4), as was pyruvate 571 μmol/L (normal 34–102), with a normal lactate/pyruvate ratio. After a 12-hour fast, AC and PC lactate and pyruvate levels were elevated similar to the initial study. Plasma amino acids were normal but a urine amino acid chromatogram showed high alanine levels. Mass spectrometry of urine organic acids indicated increased lactate 550 mg/gm Cr (normal 30–70), and 3-hydroxyisobutyrate 30 mg/gm Cr (normal 1–9).

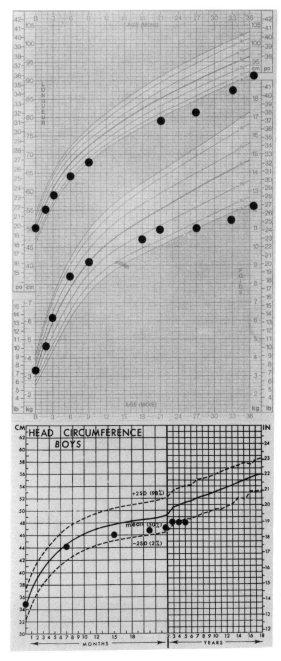

FIG. 1. Patients' height, weight, and head circumference measurements. Initially they were in the normal range but fell below the 2nd percentile by 3 years of age.

CT Scan of the brain showed mild prominence of the cerebrospinal fluid spaces with some decreased density in the periventricular white matter. An MRI scan was normal. The interictal EEG showed mild to moderate diffuse disturbance with slow immature background for his age but without epileptiform or lateralized abnormalities. Chest x-ray, EKG, abdominal ultrasound, chromosomes, ABR, SER, EMG, nerve conduction studies, and ophthalmological exam were all normal.

Treatment consisted of thiamine 50 mg and biotin 10 mg daily, carnitine 120 mg every 6 hours, sodium bicarbonate 4 ml every 6 hours, with a low carbohydrate and high fat diet. During a hemiplegic attack provoked by adenitis and fever the patient was hyperventilating and blood gas revealed a pH of 7.50; pCO_2 16 mmHg; hydrogen ion concentration 32; bicarbonate 12.7 mEq/L, base excess -7, and serum lactate of 19.7 mmol/L.

At 21 months of age a phosphorus magnetic resonance spectroscopy (MRS) of muscle showed a high intracellular inorganic phosphate with acidosis and normal brain phosphorus MRS. At 3½ years of age phosphorus MRS of muscle revealed elevated inorganic phosphate, and low phosphocreatine; inorganic phosphate ratio. Proton MRS of brain showed markedly elevated lactate with normal choline and N-acetylaspartate resonance intensities.

Assay of cultured skin fibroblast indicated pyruvate dehydrogenase complex deficiency with specific pyruvate decarboxylase El activity markedly decreased (Table 1). Pyruvate carboxylase, lipoamide dehydrogenase (E3), and dihydrolipoyl transacetylase (E3) levels were normal.

Sequencing of the PDH-El, alpha cDNA showed a guanine to adenine mutation at position 595 on the coding sequence of PDH-El alpha subunit which alters amino acid 170 from alanine to threonine in the derived amino acid sequence. Sequencing of the maternal PDH-El alpha cDNA showed only the wild type sequence. This suggests that the defect was a germ-line mutation.

DISCUSSION

This patient presented with a history of vomiting and developmental delay; investigation revealed a marked elevation of lactate and pyruvate with a normal ratio.

TABLE 1. *Results of PDHC enzyme analysis compared to controls*

Pyruvate dehydrogenase complex	Patient (mean ± SD)	Controls (mean ± SD)	Percent of controls
Pyruvate dehydrogenase: native (nmoles/ min/mg protein)	0.242 ± 0.060	1.058 ± 0.108	23
Pyruvate dehydrogenase: Dichloroacetate activated (nmoles/min/mg protein)	0.236 ± 0.037	1.190 ± 0.114	20
Pyruvate decarboxylase E1 (nmoles/hr/ mg protein)	0.07	0.65	11
Cellular lactate/pyruvate ratio	17.5 ± 1.8	21.3 ± 2.2	82

Phosphorus and proton MRS of muscle and brain showed evidence of metabolic abnormalities consistent with mitochondrial dysfunction (5,6). A deficiency of PDHC, specifically pyruvate decarboxylase El, and a point mutation of the DNA coding sequence of El subunit was identified.

Pyruvate decarboxylase (El) is one of the three main enzymes of the PDH complex. The El component is composed of alpha and beta subunits linked in a tetramere. Mutations in the gene for the El alpha subunit are located on the short end of the X chromosome at position Xp22.1 and account for the greatest majority of cases of PDHC deficiency (7). The proportion of the active enzyme in different tissues varies. In the brain the PDHC operates at about 70% of maximal activity under normal conditions and even mild deficiencies can impair brain function (8).

The clinical spectrum of PDH-El alpha deficiency is extremely varied. Brown (9) and Robinson (10) reviewed the clinical presentation in their 29 and 54 patients, respectively. The majority of patients have a prenatal onset suggested by the history of intrauterine growth retardation and cerebral dysgenesis. Agenesis of the corpus callosum, cystic lesions of the cerebral white and gray matter, basal ganglia, and brainstem are frequent findings. These patients usually die in early infancy and have a PDH-El enzyme activity of less than 15%. Other clinical features which may be associated include apneic spells, hypotonia, and seizures. Dysmorphism is not universally reported (11) but can consist of broad nasal bridge, upturned nose, micrognathia, low set posteriorly rotated ears, and simian creases.

Infants with a second phenotype of PDH-El deficiency present after a few months of age with symptoms similar to those described above in addition to ataxia, developmental delay, ophthalmoplegia, and cranial nerve palsies. These patients usually have PDH-El levels of about 20% to 35% of normal activity. Approximately one third of these children die in infancy with pathology characteristic of Leigh's syndrome.

The third group of PDH-El deficiency leads to a relatively benign syndrome with intermittent ataxia provoked by a high carbohydrate diet. Patients have residual enzyme activity in the 20% to 35% range (10). Other authors report a poor correlation between residual enzyme activity and clinical manifestations (3,9). In addition there is often heterogeneity in different tissue residual enzyme activity. De Vivo (3) reports seven children with the benign phenotype of fluctuating ataxia, post-exercise fatigue, transient paraparesis, and thiamine responsiveness. Mental and motor development was normal between episodes. All patients were males and none were reported to have intermittent hemiplegia.

In AHC specific focal abnormalities shown by neuroimaging techniques, lactic acidosis, and pathological abnormalities in muscle biopsies have not been demonstrated. A systematic study of mitochondrial respiratory chain enzymes has also not been carried out. However a study of four unrelated patients with AHC showed evidence of mitochondrial dysfunction with phosphorus MRS. All four patients had abnormally high resonance intensities for inorganic phosphate and low calculated cytosolic phosphorylation potential (2).

Our patient started to have episodes of alternating hemiplegia at 18 months of age at the upper level of the range of most patients with the syndrome of AHC. The episodes of hemiplegia in this patient occurred less frequently (about once a month) compared to most of the children with alternating hemiplegia where the spells occur with a mean frequency of 11 per month (range 2–20) (12). Although ophthalmoplegia and nystagmus have been reported in both alternating hemiplegia and PDHC deficiency (13), this child did not have any extra-ocular movement abnormalities. He also did not develop any other paroxysmal features such as dystonic attacks, choreoathetosis, or autonomic instability. The attacks in AHC are often provoked by excitement, exposure to bright light, or fatigue (12), but in this patient they were either spontaneous or triggered by intercurrent illnesses such as upper respiratory infections or gastroenteritis. Resolution of the hemiplegic attacks in AHC typically occurs after brief sleep, a pattern which was present in our patient with PDHC as well (Table 2).

The history of alternating hemiplegia in this patient with documented PDHC deficiency establishes that AHC can be a result of mitochondrial disease. This can occur despite lack of structural changes on CT or MRI. Furthermore not all patients with mitochondrial disorders have evidence of metabolic acidosis or increased serum lactate or pyruvate. In some patients there is a significant dissociation between serum and cerebral spinal fluid lactate concentration (14).

The brain is probably the organ most vulnerable to PDHC deficiency as there is barely enough enzyme activity to support maximal rates of glucose oxidation in the normal cerebrum (3,4). Excess glycolysis and lactic acid production would result from high energy demands on a brain which has a partial deficit of PDHC. A severe PDHC deficiency will cause marked chronic brain acidosis and result in neuronal death from a direct effect of the high lactate or depletion of intracellular ATP. Necrotic cystic lesions can develop in areas where there is the greatest energy requirement. However, when the PDHC deficiency is milder, the symptoms can result in transient, focal neurological symptoms, such as in the case of alternating hemiplegia when stresses such as intercurrent illness or high carbohydrate load are present. This patient demonstrates that mitochondrial dysfunction, specifically

TABLE 2. *Features of AHC in comparison to mitochondrial disorders*

	AHC	PDH-E1	Mitochondrial disease
Onset prior to 18 mo	+	+	+
Alternating hemiplegia	+	+	−
Ocular motor disorder	+	−	+
Movement disorder	+	−	+
Retardation	+	+	+
Remits with sleep	+	+	−
Provocation	Bright lights, excitement	Intercurrent illness	Intercurrent illness
Neuroimaging	−	−	+
MRS	+	+	+

PDH-E1, patient reported; +, abnormality present; −, abnormality absent.

PDH-El deficiency can result in alternating hemiplegia. Paroxysmal manifestation of PDH-El deficiency are known to occur and result in benign intermittent ataxia, but alternating hemiplegia has not been previously reported. The clinical similarity of PDH-El deficiency to AHC offers additional support that the latter may be due to mitochondrial dysfunction. A systematic evaluation of these patients with interictal and ictal blood gases, serum and CSF lactate, and pyruvate should be done. In addition analysis of mitochondrial enzymes, specifically PDHC activity with genetic studies, should be performed to identify a possible mitochondrial dysfunction which could result in AHC.

ACKNOWLEDGMENT

We thank Dr. Paul Matthews for his critical review of this chapter.

REFERENCES

1. Aicardi J. Alternating hemiplegia of childhood. *Int Pediatr* 1987;2:115–119.
2. Arnold DL, Silver K, Andermann F. Evidence for mitochondrial dysfunction in patients with alternating hemiplegia of childhood. *Ann Neurol* 1993;33:604–607.
3. De Vivo D. The expanding clinical spectrum of mitochondrial diseases. *Brain Dev* 1993;15:1–22.
4. Robinson BH, MacMillan H, Petrova Benedict R, Sherwood G. Variable clinical presentation in patients with defective El component of pyruvate dehydrogenase complex. *Pediatrics* 1987;111: 525–533.
5. Matthews PM, Allaire C, Shoubridge EA, Karpati G, Carpenter S, Arnold DL. In vivo muscle magnetic resonance spectroscopy in the clinical investigation of mitochondrial disease. *Neurology* 1991;41:114–120
6. Matthews PM, Andermann F, Silver K, Karpati G, Arnold DL. Proton MR spectroscopy characterization of differences in regional brain metabolic abnormalities in mitochondrial encephalomyopathies. *Neurology* 1993;43(12):2484–2490.
7. Brown RM, Dahl HHM, Brown GK. X-Chromosome localization of the functional gene for the El subunit of the human pyruvate dehydrogenase complex. *Genomics* 1989;4:174–181.
8. Booth RFG, Clark JB. The control of pyruvate dehydrogenase in isolated brain mitochondria. *J Neurochem* 1978;30:1003–1008.
9. Brown GK. Pyruvate dehydrogenase El deficiency. *J In Rev Metab Disorder* 1992;15:625–633.
10. Robinson BH. Lactic acidemia. In: Scriver CR. *The metabolic basis of inherited disease*, 6th ed. New York: McGraw-Hill; 1989:869–888.
11. Brown GK, Brown RM, Scholem RD, Kirby DM, Dahl HHM. The clinical and biochemical spectrum of human pyruvate dehydrogenase complex deficiency. *Ann N Y Acad Sci* 1989;573:360–368.
12. Silver K, Andermann F. Alternating hemiplegia of childhood: A study of 10 patients and results of flunarizine treatment. *Neurology* 1993;43:36–44.
13. Blass JP, Cederbaum SD, and Dunn HG. Biochemical abnormalities in Leigh's disease. *Lancet* 1976;1:1237–1238.
14. Brown GK, Haan EA, Kirby DM, et al. "Cerebral" lactic acidosis: Defects in pyruvate metabolism with profound brain damage and minimal systemic acidosis. *Eur J Pediatr* 1988;147:10–14.

Alternating Hemiplegia of Childhood, edited by
Frederick Andermann, Jean Aicardi, and Federico Vigevano,
Raven Press, Ltd., New York © 1995.

21

Recurrent Episodes of Alternating Hemiplegia and Livedo Reticularis

*Peter S. Baxter, †D. Gardner-Medwin, ‡Stuart H. Green, and
‡Celia Moss

*Department of Paediatrics, *Northern General Hospital NHS Trust,
Sheffield S5 7AU, England; †Newcastle General Hospital,
Newcastle upon Tyne NE4 6BE, England; and ‡Institute of Child Health,
University of Birmingham, Birmingham B16 8ET, England.*

Recurrent, often alternating, hemiplegia and other episodic focal neurological features can be associated with congenital livedo reticularis. The likely pathogenesis is a congenital generalized vasculopathy.

Four children have been described (1,2). Clinical details are given in Table 1. The father of one had hemiplegic migraine, but there was no other significant family history. Neurological symptoms usually began in childhood, rather than infancy, with any combination of headache, malaise, vomiting, pallor, sweatiness, confusion, focal or generalized seizures (including a dystonic element), visual spectra, hemianopia, hemisensory symptoms (including pain), dysphasia, and hemiparesis, mostly lasting a few hours to 2 days, but in one lasting up to 7 days. Attacks seemed more frequent and severe in winter and increased with age. Two developed fixed spasticity, with dementia in one and nonprogressive learning difficulties in the other. Early neuroimaging and cerebral angiography were normal but later CT and MRI scans showed cortical atrophy, with focal abnormalities. Neuropathological investigation was not performed. Anticonvulsants, antimigraine agents, antiplatelet drugs, and flunarizine were ineffective, but nifedipine reduced attack frequency and severity in two patients, while another, followed for a year, had no attacks while taking propranolol.

Alternating hemiplegia of childhood (AHC) differs from the above by an earlier age at onset, the subsequent development of dyskinesia, the normal CT findings, and the response to flunarizine. Nifedipine, a dihydropyridine, and flunarizine, a diphenylalkylamine, both reduce calcium influx through slow conducting cell membrane channels. However there are tissue and organ specific differences: for example, flunarizine probably also blocks a neuronal calcium channel, while nifedipine is a more effective systemic vasodilator.

TABLE 1. *Clinical findings in four patients with congenital vasculopathy*

Sex	Age	Onset	Episodes	Other problems	Investigations
M	21	1	2–48 hours: Infancy: staring, malaise, vomiting, confusion, and version of eyes and head Later: headache; hemisensory tingling, pain, numbness &/or "a large hand" (at first often left-sided); ±hemiparesis; ±dysphasia; ±hemianopia; ±fortification spectra; ±focal or generalized clonic seizures. Nifedipine: Marked reduction in attacks	Congenital livedo reticularis Raynaud's phenomenon; pernio vulgaris GI bleeding Bilateral glaucoma Focal hypertrophy Hypertension (age 20) Progressive bilateral spastic hemiplegia (without dystonia or dyskinesia) Progressive dementia (IQ 88, later 62)	Coagulation normal; ESR: raised in attacks Anticardiolipin IgG +ve; lupus anticoagulant, DNA, Rho, La antibodies −ve; Complement normal; DMSA scan: small right kidney; Aortography: renal artery/aortic narrowing; CT initially normal, later generalized atrophy and focal low density; Carotid arteriogram (age 4) and ultrasound carotids (age 20) normal. Skin biopsy normal
F	17	3	2–3 hours: Headache, pallor, sweating, vomiting; ±hemisensory pain, tingling (at first often left sided); ±hemiparesis; ±focal clonic seizures; unilateral neck swelling (later). Nifedipine: Hemiparesis less frequent and severe	Congenital livedo reticularis Raynaud's phenomenon + swelling of peripheries in cold; pernio vulgaris GI and mucosal bleeding Hypertension (age 11) 2° polycystic kidneys Secondary amenorrhea 2° polycystic ovaries Global learning difficulties Left dystonic and spastic hemiparesis	Late polycythemia and thrombocytopenia; ESR and, coagulation normal; Platelet responses normal; Antiphospholipid and autoantibody screen −ve; Complement normal Type IIb hyperlipidemia Cold challenge: prolonged severe response Nailbed capillaries: as in Raynaud's phenomenon CT initially normal, later cerebellar atrophy and pontine calcification MRI: lacunar infarcts Carotid arteriogram: bilateral dissections

TABLE 1. *Continued.*

Sex	Age	Onset	Episodes	Other problems	Investigations
F	8	3	7 hours to 7 days: Hemiparesis ±dysphasia; ±headache; ±pain (?where); ±hemianopia; ±focal clonic seizures; ±confusion. Nifedipine: no effect	Congenital livedo reticularis Raynaud's phenomenon; excess sweating when hot Macrocephaly Spatial, perceptual, and memory difficulties	ESR raised in attack; Coagulation normal; Autoantibody screen and complement normal; Immune complexes, lactate, cholesterol, and triglycerides slightly raised. CT: generalized atrophy with left parietal calcified hemangioma; confirmed by MRI.
F[a]	8	7	1–2 hours: Hemiparesis, vertigo, ataxia, hemianopia, impaired consciousness. Propranolol: No attacks for 1 year	Diffuse hemangiomatosis Bilateral glaucoma	Arteriography: normal

[a]Based on ref. 1.
Age, age in years at follow-up; onset: age in years at first attack.

All patients had asymmetric livedo reticularis, present from birth in three, but the age of onset is not stated for the fourth. Other problems included abnormal peripheral vascular responses to temperature change (acrocyanosis or flushing with sweating), gastrointestinal and mucosal bleeding, glaucoma, local tissue hypertrophy, and, in two patients followed to adulthood, hypertension and renal involvement. Large vessel disease also occurred, with carotid dissections in one patient and aortic, femoral, and renal arterial narrowing in another.

The distinctive feature of these children was the skin rash. Livedo reticularis describes a network pattern of blue-red discoloration of the skin. It is a nonspecific sign of impaired cutaneous circulation, either due to disease of dermal arterioles, capillaries, or venules, or due to hyperviscosity (3). It resembles cutis marmorata, the mottling seen in children in cold conditions that reflects the venous drainage system, but does not completely disappear with warming. Confusingly, in some of the European literature the term livedo racemosa describes the former and livedo reticularis the latter. When present at or soon after birth, congenital livedo reticularis can also be called cutis marmorata-telangiectasia congenita (or telangiectatica congenita), congenital generalized phlebectasia, or cutis marmorata congenita universalis, among other terms.

Congenital livedo is not usually associated with any other problems. It can be exacerbated by cold, emotion, and activity. In most cases it fades during childhood, but there may be dermatological (port wine stain, ulceration), soft tissue (localized hypertrophy or atrophy), ocular (glaucoma), and neurological complications (seizures, developmental delay) (4). In this it resembles other congenital vasculopathies such as the Sturge-Weber and Klippel-Trenaunay-Weber syndromes. The Divry-van Bogaert syndrome is the association of congenital livedo with progressive dementia, seizures, pyramidal and extrapyramidal features, starting in early adulthood. Five patients have been described, three familial. Autopsies show a predominantly venous noncalcified corticomeningeal angiomatosis, with fibrous degeneration of vessel walls, scattered cortical infarcts, and degeneration/demyelination of the white matter (diffuse meningocerebral angiomatosis and leucoencephalopathy). Similar neurological and neuropathological features have been described in two other patients with adult onset livedo and in five children without livedo, four familial (5). The distinguishing feature is the presence of leukoencephalopathy on neuroimaging.

In adults, recurrent strokes, migraine, and other forms of cerebrovascular disease are a well-recognized complication of acquired livedo reticularis. The association is often called Sneddon's syndrome. Systemic lupus erythematosus and the antiphospholipid antibody syndromes are prominent causes, together with other generalized vasculopathies (6,7). Patients often have other problems such as Raynaud's phenomenon, hypertension, and peripheral thromboses. The skin appearance is often more striking before neurological exacerbations. Endarteritis obliterans and other causes of vascular obstruction are the most common pathological finding. Treatment with antiplatelet drugs or immunosuppressants is unsatisfactory. There is no report on the effect of nifedipine. However Sneddon's syndrome has not been described in children and systemic lupus erythematosus more commonly causes seizures, psychosis, or chorea (8).

Neurological syndromes with livedo reticularis mostly seem to result from generalized vasculopathies. The latter can be divided into structural, with histological abnormalities such as vasculitis, endarteritis obliterans, malformations, etc., or functional, without histological change, which includes hyperviscosity. The investigations of the patients in Table 1 suggest a functional defect, with later structural involvement of large arteries. In one, skin biopsy with particular examination of deep and superficial dermal vessels was normal. Blood viscosity and ESR were normal at first, but the ESR was later raised during attacks. Apart from anticardiolipin antibodies in one individual, immunological investigations were normal. In two there were mild abnormalities of blood lipids. However, in one, a cold challenge (immersion of the hand in iced water for 2 minutes) evoked an abnormal response, with persisting pain, swelling, vasospasm, and thrombocytopenia 90 minutes later. Better understanding of the physiology of the endothelium and other components of blood vessels and the role of paracrine regulators such as endothelin or nitrous oxide is needed to explain the cause and to design more effective treatment, but nifedipine and adequate clothing and warmth may help.

ACKNOWLEDGMENT

We thank Dr. Brett, Professor Casaer, Dr. Hockaday, and Professor Levin for their help with these patients

REFERENCES

1. van Emde Boas W, Barth PG. Basilar artery migraine in a seven year old girl with atypical Sturge Weber syndrome. Transient brainstem dysfunction and hemiparesis documented by EEG and video. *Presented to European Federation of Child Neurology Societies.* Siena, Italy; 1985.
2. Baxter P, Gardner-Medwin D, Green SH, Moss C. Congenital livedo reticularis and recurrent stroke-like episodes. *Dev Med Child Neurol* 1993;35:917–921.
3. Quimby, SR, Perry HO. Livedo reticularis and cerebrovascular accidents. *J Am Acad Dermatol* 1980; 3:377–383.
4. Winter RM, Baraitser M. Cutis marmorata—telangiectasia congenita. In: *Multiple congenital anomalies. A diagnostic compendium.* London: Chapman and Hall Medical; 1991:146.
5. Vonsattel J-PG, Hedley-Whyte T. Diffuse meningocerebral angiomatosis and leucoencephalopathy. In: Toole JF, ed. *Vascular diseases Part III, Handbook of Clinical Neurology;* 1989:55:317–323
6. Bruyn RPM. Sneddon's syndrome. In: Toole JF, ed., *Vascular diseases Part III, Handbook of clinical neurology;* 1989:55:401–410
7. Pope JM, Canny CLB, Bell DA. Cerebral ischaemic events associated with endocarditis, retinal vascular disease and lupus anticoagulant. *Am J Med* 1991;90:299–309.
8. Shergy WJ, Kredich DW, Pisetsky DS. The relationship of anticardiolipin antibodies to disease manifestations in pediatric systemic lupus erythematosus. *J Rheumatol* 1988;15:1389–1394.

Alternating Hemiplegia of Childhood, edited by
Frederick Andermann, Jean Aicardi, and Federico Vigevano,
Raven Press, Ltd., New York © 1995.

22

Familial Hemiplegic Migraine with Altered Consciousness Followed by Peduncular Hallucinosis:

Migraine Coma as a Disorder of Brain Energy Metabolism and Possible Relevance to Alternating Hemiplegia of Childhood

Benjamin G. Zifkin*, Douglas L. Arnold,
Frederick Andermann, Eva Andermann

*Department of Neurology and Neurosurgery, McGill University, Montreal Neurological
Hospital and Institute, 3801 University Street, Montreal, Quebec H3A 2B4, Canada,
Department of Neurological Sciences, Hôpital du Sacré Coeur, de Montréal.

In 1980 (1), we reported a mother and son with hemiplegic migraine, nystagmus, and tremor, and suggested that the findings were not related to migrainous ischemia but to a system degeneration inherited with the familial hemiplegic migraine (FHM). Since then, these patients have developed new symptoms, and more is known about unusual syndromes thought to be related to migraine, notably migraine coma (2) and alternating hemiplegia. Further investigations of both subjects suggest hypotheses about the origins of these syndromes.

PATIENT 1

This woman developed alternating hemiplegia with severe headache at age 12, after a fall on ice in which she struck the back of her head. She was said to be paralyzed for weeks afterwards. Hemiplegic migraines occurred about twice monthly, related to menstruation, stress or fatigue, but later became less frequent. Tremor similar to essential tremor developed in her twenties. Neuro-ophthalmologic examinations by the same consultant over 15 years have documented coarse gaze-paretic nystagmus, impairment of optokinetic nystagmus, and failure of fixation suppression of the vestibulo-ocular reflex. Over several years the hemiplegic episodes have changed. Propranolol and pizotyline have reduced the frequency of attacks, but have not eliminated them.

Since 1982, she has been admitted three times to the Montreal Neurological Hospital with progressive headache of unilateral onset and contralateral weakness or numbness, left or right. No specific triggering factors could be identified. In 1989 and 1982, these were associated with somnolence, confusion, and in the former case, fever to 39°C and neck stiffness with aphasia and right hemiplegia. She became more alert over 2 days but as each episode cleared, developed well-formed visual hallucinations such as silent small white dogs running around her room, people, or objects (a horse and a tree). These began with recovery of her usual level of consciousness. She was agitated or confused at their onset, but soon realized their hallucinatory nature with increasing alertness and was perplexed by them. These hallucinations, suggestive of peduncular hallucinosis, resolved over 1–2 days without neuroleptic drugs. There has been no lasting neurologic deficit following her attacks. There has been some progression of head and arm tremor over nearly 15 years, but it continues to resemble essential tremor without parkinsonian, dystonic, or dyskinetic features. The eye movement disorder has not progressed.

CT scans and MRI brain imaging have been normal as have visual, auditory, and median and posterior tibial somatosensory evoked responses obtained after recovery from the hallucinosis. Lumbar punctures have been sterile, with normal CSF protein, glucose, and IgG during the headaches. No oligoclonal bands were found. The CSF VDRL has been negative. In 1989, there were 6×10^9 lymphocytes per litre in association with fever and stiff neck. Serial EEGs during attacks have shown diffuse delta activity which has been paroxysmal at times. There has often been predominance of abnormal slow wave activity contralateral to the weakness or numbness, but this has not been invariable. The EEG improved with clinical improvement, and no epileptiform activity has been recorded either with sensorimotor symptoms or with hallucinations. In 1982 and 1989, serum aspartate and alanine aminotransferase levels were within normal limits several times. In 1992, alanine aminotransferase and lactate dehydrogenase were slightly elevated. Karyotype was normal 46,XX. Because of suspected mitochondrial encephalopathy, further investigations were performed in 1989 and 1992 (Table 1).

PATIENT 2 (SON OF PATIENT 1)

About 6 weeks after an automobile accident at age 12, in which he did not lose consciousness, he developed sudden weakness and numbness of the left leg. One hour later he had severe headache lasting 30 minutes. Attacks then occurred in groups, several in one week followed by asymptomatic periods of several weeks. He recalled tremor of the head and left arm from age 12 as well. An EEG performed during that time was reportedly normal. He was given phenytoin without any change in the pattern or frequency of attacks. At age 18 years in 1973, he was of low average intelligence, with head and arm tremor resembling essential tremor,

TABLE 1. *Summary of investigations in patients 1 and 2*[a]

Test	Date	Patient 1	Patient 2
Skin and muscle biopsy	1989	Skin and eccrine cell mitochondria normal. Muscle fibers with very thin subsarcolemmal crescents. No ragged red fibers or mitochondrial excess	
Serum lactate	1989	0.7 and 0.8 mmol/l (1–1.8) during hospitalization	
Serum lactate (fasting)	1992	1.2 mmol/l (asymptomatic)	0.7 mmol/l (asymptomatic)
Serum lactate (fasting)	1992	1.8 and 1.6 mmol/l following recovery from hallucinosis	
Serum pyruvate (fasting)	1992	0.04 mmol/l (0.03–0.10) (asymptomatic)	0.05 mmol/l (asymptomatic)
Serum pyruvate (fasting)	1992	0.15 and 0.21 mmol/l following recovery from hallucinosis	
Serum alanine (fasting)	1992	466 μmol/l (less than 500 μmol/l) when asymptomatic	600 μmol/l (asymptomatic)
Serum alanine (fasting)	1992	719 μmol/l following recovery from hallucinosis	
CSF lactate	1992	2.2 mmol/l (less than 3.0 mmol/l) following recovery from hallucinosis	
CSF pyruvate	1992	0.13 mmol/l (less than 0.19 mmol/l) following recovery from hallucinosis	
^{18}F-FDG PET	1992	Symmetric 30–40% reduction in cerebral glucose utilization rate indicating diffuse reduction of cerebral blood flow.	
^{31}Phosphorus MRS of gastrocnemius muscle after recovery from attacks.	1985		Normal
	1989	Elevated inorganic phosphate, borderline high phosphocreatine, low ADP. Similar results in 1992.	Normal
^{1}Hydrogen MRS of brain	1992	Suggestive of neuronal loss. Lactate not elevated (after recovery).	

[a]Some values were obtained twice during the same hospitalization. Reference ranges are in parentheses.

FDG-PET, fluorodeoxyglucose positron emission tomography; MRS, magnetic resonance spectroscopy.

and nystagmus. The EEG was normal, and an electronystagmogram recorded low amplitude right spontaneous and positional nystagmus, though he did not cooperate for a full study. The audiogram was normal. He was given propranolol, 40 mg t.i.d. Since then, he has continued to have attacks, coming to the hospital only when the weakness is severe or prolonged. He has been admitted in 1974, 1985, and 1989 with headache, hemiplegia, somnolence, and aphasia when the hemiplegia was right-sided. In 1974, carotid arteriography during an episode of right hemiplegia showed vasospasm of sylvian branches of the left middle cerebral artery. He has had one documented episode of confusion, agitation, and formed visual hallucinations suggesting peduncular hallucinosis during recovery of normal alertness. During this period he was also described as intermittently catatonic. In 1989, he also had fever of 39°C and leukocytosis, with normal CSF protein, glucose, and cell count. Attacks last several days to a week and have occurred despite pizotyline and propranolol. The tremor and eye movement disorder remain unchanged. His brain MRI and CT scans have been normal, as have been visual, auditory, and somatosensory evoked responses. Further investigations are summarized in Table 1.

DISCUSSION

The family members reported here appear to suffer from migraine coma (2) characterized by stupor or coma in the setting of severe FHM, with fever and CSF pleocytosis. Fitzsimons and Wolfenden reported lateralized cerebral edema, psychotic features on emergence from coma, and cerebellar ataxia becoming persistent and associated with cerebellar atrophy following repeated attacks. Transmission from a father to sons and probably to a daughter was compatible with autosomal dominant rather than maternal inheritance. Extensive biochemical investigations disclosed only transient and inconsistent elevations of plasma alanine with normal activity of pyruvate dehydrogenase (PDH) and carboxylase, and phosphoenolpyruvate carboxylase in cultured skin fibroblasts, and normal muscle biopsy. One subject with a normal random pyruvate level had elevated serum pyruvate while ill.

FHM is a rare disorder distinct from hemiplegic migraine or classical migraine with lateralized weakness (3,4). Several earlier cases of FHM with altered consciousness and psychotic symptoms without evidence of migraine-related brain infarcts to account for them have also been reported. No biochemical evidence is available for these families, but the clinical pattern is strikingly similar to the cases described here. In addition to the cases reviewed by Fitzsimons and Wolfenden, Gastaut et al. (5) reported a mother and son with fever, meningeal signs, and prominent drowsiness accompanying hemiplegic migraine. O'Hare et al. (6) described FHM, often precipitated by trivial head trauma, associated with drowsiness followed by agitation and hallucinations in the index patient, his male cousin, and his aunt who first came to medical attention at age 78 but who had had attacks of hemiplegia, confusion, disturbed consciousness, and hallucinations since her youth without lasting deficits. The index patient also had fever and stiff neck with his attacks. Feely et al. (7) extended these observations over four generations and nine subjects with FHM, eight of whom had acute confusion or psychosis with auditory or visual hallucinations, some with paranoid delusions, after the return of alertness. The history again suggested autosomal dominant inheritance. The hallucinations in our patients suggested peduncular hallucinosis, as originally described by Lhermitte (8), often but not invariably associated with midbrain lesions. The pathologic anatomy has been reviewed by McKee et al. (9). The predilection for small animals, which appears to be shared with Korsakoff's psychosis, remains unexplained.

Migraine coma can be lethal. A patient with FHM presenting with fever, neck stiffness, drowsiness, and hemiplegia developed convulsions and coma. Respiratory arrest followed and a persistent vegetative state ended with death from intercurrent infection 4 months later. Autopsy showed no infarction of respiratory centers or other significant brainstem lesions, and the authors noted that it was "curious that an ischemic insult of this . . . severity may leave no pathological trace of damage in the appropriate site (10). The family described by Fitzsimons and Wolfenden (2) reported deaths from "meningitis" after trivial head injury in 1915 and 1926, and one of their patients survived respiratory arrest during an attack. Migraine coma was also lethal in a 12-year-old with FHM reported by Mallet et al. (11).

Biochemical investigations have not been consistent but a pattern of elevated plasma alanine and elevated pyruvate has been seen in our subjects and others, with a rise from normal levels to much higher values following an attack. Ammonia levels were not increased. Lactic acidemia has been sought but never found, and MRS performed following recovery in one of our two patients, though abnormal, confirmed that brain lactate was not increased. The increased alanine levels, observed in asymptomatic as well as ill subjects, most likely reflect tissue pyruvate accumulation and transamination to alanine. Most circulating alanine arises from muscle and the contribution of the relatively small brain tissue volume must be small at resting conditions. The high alanine levels between attacks suggest a subclinical disturbance of pyruvate metabolism in muscle. Our biopsied patient also had a nonspecific abnormality of muscle mitochondria not seen in previously reported patients suggesting a defect that may be more severe or more widespread and which may explain the inconsistent results of plasma levels from family to family. Muscle ^{31}phosphorus MRS showed elevated inorganic phosphate twice over 3 years in one of our patients, also suggesting a subtle defect of energy metabolism. In our subjects, maternal transmission cannot be excluded, but male to male and male to female transmission is well documented and is most consistent with autosomal dominant inheritance, excluding disorders of mitochondrial DNA. Lactate/pyruvate ratios have been more consistent with a disorder of PDH than with a respiratory chain disorder and normal ammonia levels are against a urea cycle disorder.

We believe that migraine coma is a disorder of pyruvate metabolism which is diffuse but whose clinical manifestations are confined to the brain. Although there is indirect evidence of pyruvate excess, it is not a typical form of PDH deficiency clinically or biochemically. The relation of FHM to this disorder is not clear. Families with FHM but without migraine coma have been described (4) but the two appear to be inherited together often in this rare disorder. It has been suggested that brain PDH has specific functions notably in cholinergic neurons in which it is selectively concentrated and where it provides acetyl-CoA for acetylcholine synthesis (12). Pathophysiologic levels of surrounding Ca^{2+} reduce PDH activity in rat brain mitochondria (13), and added Ca^{2+} reduces acetyl-CoA in synaptosomal mitochondria (14). The ischemia associated with the migraine attack may trigger clinical expression of the defect in migraine coma by widespread exposure of compromised but adequately functioning brain mitochondria to an intolerable calcium ion concentration that leads to diffuse transient mitochondrial failure combined with a more specific system failure of cholinergic neurons. More severe impairment, which may be due to factors such as duration and distribution of ischemia, degree, and extent of the metabolic defect, or exacerbation of mitochondrial dysfunction with reperfusion, may lead to localized or diffuse brain-specific cell loss; or cell loss in selectively vulnerable, possibly cholinergic cell groups, and may be responsible for fixed or progressive deficits seen between migraine attacks without producing macroscopic lesions.

Alternating hemiplegia of childhood (AHC) has often been related to migraine. It is however more severe and more complex than usual childhood migraine, with both intermittent and lasting clinical features not typical of migraine. Dystonia or nystagmus often precede the development of hemiplegic attacks, and there are typically both paroxysmal (nystagmus, tachycardia, sweating, mydriasis, dystonia) and fixed deficits (ataxia, chorea, mental retardation) (15–17). Patients with AHC would not be expected to reproduce, but one family with autosomal dominant AHC has been reported (18). AHC has been found in both PDH deficiency (see Chapter 20) and in the syndrome of mitochondrial encephalopathy, lactic acidosis, and strokes (MELAS) (19) both of which involve defects in mitochondrial energy production, though AHC is not typical of MELAS. AHC patients do not have strokes or basal ganglia calcifications (20), acidosis, elevated serum pyruvate or lactate, or ragged red muscle fibers (21), but muscle MRS in four patients reported by D.L. Arnold et al. (29a) showed a significant increase of inorganic phosphate in all, suggesting a subtle disturbance in energy metabolism.

The calcium channel blocker flunarizine has been studied in AHC (15,16,22) and several drugs of this class are useful in migraine, including hemiplegic migraine (23). These drugs are also effective in preventing or reducing the toxic effects of Ca^{2+} on mitochondrial morphology and function in ischemic and reperfused heart (24–27). All antimigraine calcium channel blockers act at voltage-dependent L-type dihydropyridine-sensitive Ca^{2+} channels (28) but multiple voltage-dependent channel types have recently been identified, not affected by dihydropyridines and therefore probably not by clinically available Ca^{2+} channel blockers (29,30). This may explain the incomplete though helpful results obtained with these drugs in AHC and in complicated or hemiplegic migraine (15,16,22,23). It is noteworthy that propranolol and pizotyline, which are not Ca^{2+} channel blockers, did not prevent migraine coma in our patients.

Migraine coma and AHC may both be due to genetic defects of mitochondrial energy production, but the metabolic defect in these two disorders may be different. Findings in migraine coma are compatible with pyruvate excess and inadequate acetyl-CoA production. MRS and muscle biopsy results are nonspecifically abnormal, not excluding mitochondrial disorders, but if both syndromes are autosomally inherited, and the evidence for autosomal dominant transmission in migraine coma is strong, then abnormalities of proteins encoded in mitochondrial DNA are excluded for both. The defect or defects could involve control of PDH function, assembly, or structure.

Rust et al. suggest that AHC may be related to a novel abnormality of the Krebs cycle (31) and have also suggested on the basis of ^{1}H MRS that migrainous hemiplegia results from a metabolic mechanism rather than from ischemia (32). Montagna et al. (33) have suggested that migraine is a disorder of brain oxidative metabolism, and found metabolic defects in [31]phosphorus MRS of muscle in eight patients with complicated migraine or migraine-related strokes (34). Twelve subjects with classic migraine studied between attacks had normal [31]phosphorus MRS of resting gastrocnemius muscle but there was MRS evidence of abnormal mitochondrial function without clinical muscle disease in nine cases (35).

Systematic investigation of migraine coma and AHC patients, and their families, for hyperalaninemia, hyperpyruvicacidemia, and abnormalities of PDH function both between and during attacks seems worthwhile, as does brain and muscle MRS. We had originally suggested that the syndrome we reported (1) represented a system degeneration inherited with FHM, but it seems more compatible with a familial disorder of energy metabolism. The abnormalities found in an apparently sporadic case of hemiplegic migraine without migraine coma (30) and in other cases of migraine suggest that all FHM and possibly all migraine with lateralized neurological deficit is not migraine at all as it is commonly understood, but instead a disorder of brain energy production. This is not incompatible with recent theories of a primary role for the endothelial cell in the pathogenesis of all migraine (36), and offers an explanation for the striking consequences of ischemia seen in migraine coma.

CONCLUSION

A mother and son with FHM, nystagmus, and tremor developed episodes of hemiplegic migraine and stupor, at times with meningeal signs. With recovery of consciousness, they became agitated and developed hallucinations suggesting peduncular hallucinosis. Attacks were not prevented by propranolol or pizotyline. Blood alanine levels were high, and pyruvate increased during an attack. Lactate was not increased in blood or on ^{1}H brain magnetic resonance spectroscopy. This syndrome has been described as migraine coma. We believe that it is caused by an autosomal dominant defect in cerebral energy metabolism inherited with familial hemiplegic migraine and possibly related to disturbance of PDH activity. There are similarities between migraine coma and AHC. Both may reflect brain mitochondrial failure with toxic calcium ion influx as a common pathway but the cause of the defect may not be the same.

ACKNOWLEDGMENTS

Alanine levels were performed by Ms. Carol Clow and staff of the DeBelle Laboratory for Biochemical Genetics, Montreal Children's Hospital. Dr. Kenneth Silver provided helpful advice. Dr. T. H. Kirkham performed the neuro-ophthalmological examinations.

REFERENCES

1. Zifkin B, Andermann E, Andermann F, Kirkham T. An autosomal dominant syndrome of hemiplegic migraine, nystagmus, and tremor. *Ann Neurol* 1980;8:329–332.
2. Fitzsimons RB, Wolfenden WH. Migraine coma. Meningitic migraine with cerebral oedema associated with a new form of autosomal dominant cerebellar ataxia. *Brain* 1985;108:555–577.
3. Whitty CW. Familial hemiplegic migraine. *J Neurol Neurosurg Psychiatry* 1953;16:172–177.
4. Glista GG, Mellinger JF, Rooke ED. Familial hemiplegic migraine. *Mayo Clin Proc* 1975;50:307–311.
5. Gastaut JL, Yermenos E, Bonnefoy M, Cros D. Familial hemiplegic migraine: EEG and CT scan study of two cases. *Ann Neurol* 1981;10:392–395.
6. O'Hare JA, Feely MP, Callaghan N. Clinical aspects of familial hemiplegic migraine in two families. *Irish Med J* 1981;74:291–295.
7. Feely MP, O'Hare JA, Veale D, Callaghan N. Episodes of acute confusion or psychosis in familial hemiplegic migraine. *Acta Neurol Scand* 1982;65:369–375.
8. Lhermitte J. Syndrome de la calotte du pédoncule cérébral. Les troubles psychosensoriels dans les lésions du mésocéphale. *Rev Neurol* 1922;38:1359–1365.
9. McKee AC, Levine DN, Kowall NW, Richardson EP Jr. Peduncular hallucinosis associated with isolated infarction of the substantia nigra pars reticulata. *Ann Neurol* 1990;27:500–504.
10. Neligan P, Harriman DG, Pearce J. Respiratory arrest in familial hemiplegic migraine: a clinical and neuropathological study. *BMJ* 1977;2:732–734.
11. Mallet R, Sterba S, Ribière M, Labrune B. Migraine hémiplégique familiale. *Ann Pédiatr (Paris)* 1968;36–37:519–525.
12. Sheu KFR, Szabo P, Ko LW, Hinman LM. Abnormalities of pyruvate dehydrogenase complex in brain disease. *Ann N Y Acad Sci* 1989;573:378–391.
13. Lai JCK, Sheu KFR. Calcium loading of brain mitochondria alters pyruvate dehydrogenase complex activity and flux. *Ann N Y Acad Sci* 1989;573:423–425.
14. Bielaczyk H, Szutowicz A. Evidence for the regulatory function of synaptoplasmic acetyl Co-A in acetylcholine synthesis in nerve endings. *Biochem J* 1989;262:377–380.
15. Alvarez Gomez MJ, Narbona Garcia J, Barona Zamora P. Alternating hemiplegia. Partial effectiveness of treatment with flunarizine. *Neurologia* 1992;7:116–119.
16. Casaer P. Flunarizine in alternating hemiplegia in childhood. An international study in 12 children. *Neuropediatrics* 1987;18:191–195.
17. Krägeloh I, Aicardi J. Alternating hemiplegia in infants: report of five cases. *Dev Med Child Neurol* 1980;22:784–791.
18. Mikati M, Ozelius L, Breakfield X, et al. Linkage analysis in autosomal-dominant alternating hemiplegia of childhood. *Ann Neurol* 1992;32:451 (abst).
19. Matsuzaki M, Izumi T, Ebato K, et al. Hypothalamic GH deficiency and gelastic seizures in a 10-year-old girl with MELAS. *No To Hattatsu* 1991;23:411–416.
20. Matthews PM, Tampieri D, Berkovic SF, et al. Magnetic resonance imaging shows specific abnormalities in the MELAS syndrome. *Neurology* 1991;41:1043–1046.

21. DiMauro S, Bonilla E, Lombes A, et al. Mitochondrial encephalomyopathies. *Neurol Clin* 1990;8: 483–506.
22. Silver K, Andermann F. Alternating hemiplegia of childhood: a study of 10 patients and results of flunarizine treatment. *Neurology* 1993;43(1):36–41.
23. Greenberg DA. Calcium channel antagonists and the treatment of migraine. *Clin Neuropharmacol* 1986;9:311–328.
24. Hugtenburg JG, Van Voorst MJ, Van Marle J, et al. The influence of nifedipine and mioflazine on mitochondrial calcium overload in normoxic and ischaemic guinea-pig hearts. *Eur J Pharmacol* 1990;178:71–78.
25. Zografos P, Watts JA. Shifts in calcium in ischemic and reperfused rat hearts: a cytochemical and morphometric study of the effects of diltiazem. *Am J Cardiovasc Pathol* 1990;3:155–165.
26. Dunlap ED, Matlib MA, Millard RW. Protection of regional mechanics and mitochondrial oxidative phosphorylation by amlodipine in transiently ischemic myocardium. *Am J Cardiol* 1989;64:84I–91I.
27. Ferrari R, Boraso A, Condorelli E, et al. Protective effects of gallopamil against ischemia and reperfusion damage. *Z Kardiol* 1989;78 (Suppl 5):1–11.
28. Greenberg DA. Calcium channels and calcium channel antagonists. *Ann Neurol* 1987;21:317–330.
29. Chad J. Inactivation of calcium channels. *Comp Biochem Physiol* 1989;93:95–105.
29a. Arnold DL, Silver K, Andermann F. Evidence for mitochondrial dysfunction in patients with alternating hemiplegia of childhood. *Ann Neurol* 1993;33:604–607.
30. Aosaki T, Kasai H. Characterization of two kinds of high-voltage-activated Ca-channel currents in chick sensory neurons. Differential sensitivity to dihydropyridines and omega-conotoxin GVIA. *Pflügers Arch* 1989;414:150–156.
31. Rust RS, Thomas A, Zupanc ML, Bianco JA, Turski P. ^{1}H volume localized in vivo magnetic resonance spectroscopy and single-photon emission computed tomography in alternating hemiplegia. *Ann Neurol* 1992;32:452 (abst).
32. Rust RS, Thomas AM, Chun RWM, Brown D, Turski P. Multidimensional phase-contrast angiography and ^{1}H-MR spectroscopy in the evaluation of hemiplegic migraine. *Ann Neurol* 1992;32: 485 (abst).
33. Montagna P, Sacquegna T, Cortelli P, Lugaresi E. Migraine as a defect of brain oxidative metabolism [Letter]. *J Neurol* 1989;236:124–125.
34. Barbiroli B, Montagna P, Cortelli P, et al. Complicated migraine studied by phosphorus magnetic resonance spectroscopy. *Cephalagia* 1990;10:263–272.
35. Barbiroli B, Montagna P, Cortelli P, et al. Abnormal brain and muscle energy metabolism shown by ^{31}P magnetic resonance spectroscopy in patients affected by migraine with aura. *Neurology* 1992;42:1209–1214.
36. Appenzeller O. Pathogenesis of migraine. *Med Clin North Am* 1991;75:763–789.

Alternating Hemiplegia of Childhood:
Attempts at Treatment

Alternating Hemiplegia of Childhood, edited by
Frederick Andermann, Jean Aicardi, and Federico Vigevano,
Raven Press, Ltd., New York © 1995.

23

The Treatment of Alternating Hemiplegia of Childhood with Flunarizine

Experience with 17 Patients

Marie Bourgeois and *Jean Aicardi

*Department of Pediatrics, Hôpital des Enfants Malades, 149 rue de Sèvres,
75743 Paris Cedex 15, France; and *Institute of Child Health, University of London,
Mecklenburgh Square, London WC1N 2AP, England.*

Flunarizine has been shown to be effective in the treatment of alternating hemiplegia of childhood (AHC) (1,3) although complete control of attacks is only exceptionally (4), if ever, achieved. Both Casaer et al. (1) and Silver and Andermann (2) found that flunarizine therapy reduced the duration and severity of hemiplegic attacks but only infrequently diminished their frequency. We report our experience with flunarizine treatment in 17 children with AHC. The duration of treatment varied from 18 months to 9 years (average 5.2 years). Treatment was started at 1 year of age in one child, between 1 and 2 years of age in three, between 2 and 5 years in ten, and over 5 years in three patients. The dose used varied between 5 and 20 mg, most children receiving 10 mg daily. In only one child was treatment discontinued because of lack of efficacy.

RESULTS

In only one patient was the frequency of attacks significantly decreased (by more than 50%). Nine of the children had a significant decrease in the severity and duration of their hemiplegic attacks whose average duration was reduced from up to several days to a few hours. Furthermore, the degree of weakness was less profound and some use of the affected side remained possible. The frequency of attacks, on the other hand, did not change significantly, the average interval between attacks being less than 10 days in 12 patients and between 10 and 15 days in five. In five cases, there was no or only an insignificant improvement.

In several cases, flunarizine did not prevent extension of hemiplegic weakness to the opposite side. Quadriplegic episodes, that represent the most severe manifestation of AHC, do not seem to be prevented by the drug. In two children the frequency and intensity of bilateral episodes did not seem to be influenced by the treatment. In three children treated between 1 and 2 years of age, severe bilateral attacks were frequent and prolonged.

Flunarizine did not appear to be effective against other paroxysmal manifestations of AHC, especially dystonic attacks and paroxysmal ocular movement abnormalities. However, these manifestations usually disappear before 6–10 years of age whether the patients are treated or not, so any therapeutic effect is hard to prove.

There was no obvious difference in outcome between patients treated early (1–2 years) in the course and those who received flunarizine later (6–9.5 years).

A dose of 5 mg per day was as effective as higher doses in one patient and a dose of 7.5 mg in one other. For most children, a dose of 10 mg seemed to be necessary. Four children who received doses of 15 and 20 mg daily did not demonstrate further improvement. The positive effects of the drug were possibly less clear after the first 2 or 3 years of therapy in eight cases.

No severe side-effect was observed in any patient. In particular, no extrapyramidal symptom or sign was ever found. The parents of three patients thought that the frequency and intensity of tonic/dystonic seizures increased at doses in excess of 7.5 mg. In five other children, increased irritability and excitation were thought to be associated with flunarizine therapy.

A combination of flunarizine with other drugs, especially anticonvulsant agents, was used in several cases. The parents of four children who received diazepam and those of two patients who received phenytoin in addition to flunarizine believed that the combination was more effective than either agent alone.

COMMENTS

Our experience with flunarizine in the treatment of AHC is similar to that of other investigators (1,2). We also found that any effect of the drug was mainly on duration and severity of attacks rather than on their frequency. Our results have been overall relatively disappointing as 7 of 17 (41%) of our patients showed no significant response. Perhaps more importantly, we did not find any obvious positive effect on the occurrence and severity of bilateral attacks. Those are often associated with prolonged, and perhaps partly irreversible, deterioration so their prevention is clearly desirable.

We have not observed any dramatic improvements in the long-term outcome of children treated early in the disease, even though partial efficacy on the hemiplegic attacks was demonstrated. However, this is not a comparative study and no definitive statement regarding the prevention of cognitive and neurologic deterioration can be made.

The short-term efficacy of flunarizine on the hemiplegic episodes of AHC has been demonstrated in one controlled study (1). The mode of action remains un-known. Interestingly, although flunarizine has a very long half-life with consequent build-up of blood levels over several weeks (5), the effect on hemiplegias was usually almost immediate. Likewise, the effect decreased rapidly in those patients for whom a drug holiday of 5 days was prescribed at the end of each month of treatment, suggesting that the mode of action is not entirely dependent on drug levels.

Further studies of flunarizine therapy for AHC are indicated. A search for more effective agents is also warranted, as it appears that flunarizine is only partially effective and may not prevent the long-term consequences of AHC.

REFERENCES

1. Casaer P. Flunarizine in alternating hemiplegia in childhood. An international study of 12 children. *Neuropediatrics* 1987;18:191–195.
2. Silver K, Andermann F. Alternating hemiplegia of childhood: a study of 10 patients and results of flunarizine treatment. *Neurology* 1993;43:36–41.
3. Curatolo P. Cusmai R. Drugs for alternating hemiplegic migraine. *Lancet* 1984;2:980.
4. Casaer P, Azou M. Flunarizine in alternating hemiplegia in childhood. *Lancet* 1984;2:579.
5. Snyder S, Reynolds I. Calcium antagonist drugs. *N Engl J Med* 1985;313:995–1002.

Alternating Hemiplegia of Childhood, edited by
Frederick Andermann, Jean Aicardi, and Federico Vigevano,
Raven Press, Ltd., New York © 1995.

24

Alternating Hemiplegia of Childhood: Treatment with Flunarizine

Kenneth Silver and *Frederick Andermann

*Department of Neurology and Neurosurgery, McGill University, Montreal Children's Hospital, Montreal, Quebec H3H 1P3, Canada; and *Montreal Neurological Hospital and Institute, 3801 University Street, Montreal, Quebec H3A 2B4, Canada.*

The main thrust of treatment of alternating hemiplegia of childhood (AHC) has been with antiepileptic and migraine preventive drugs. Seven patients were initially diagnosed by us and others as having epilepsy and treated with single or multiple anticonvulsants, including phenobarbital, primidone, carbamazepine, valproic acid, diazepam, clonazepam, lorazepam, and acetazolamide without effect on the hemiplegic attacks. Four (1,2,7,9) were treated with phenytoin, without control of their attacks but attempts to discontinue this medication resulted in worsening of the hemiplegic events in three. Treatment with antimigranous prophylactic agents such as propranolol, methysergide, and pizotyline, did not result in improvement in the frequency or severity of hemiplegic attacks.

Casaer and Azou (1) reported a child whose attacks ceased after treatment with flunarizine, a calcium channel blocker. To further characterize the response to flunarizine we describe nine patients who have been treated for up to 5 years (2).

METHODS

In a retrospective study, the frequency, duration, and associated symptoms of the hemiplegic attacks were recorded in the affected patients. In an open-label study they were treated with flunarizine. The parents were requested to record the frequency, duration, and symptoms associated with the attacks during a control period and in response to flunarizine. The patients were treated with this calcium channel blocker for a mean of 2.7 years (0.5 to 5 years) with an average dose of 12.8 mg per day (range 5 to 25 mg). In 7 of the 9 who participated in this trial there was considerable reduction in the duration of attacks, by 85% overall (Fig. 2). In patients 1 and 4 attack duration was unchanged during treatment. In only one child was there

TREATMENT WITH FLUNARIZINE (N=9)
PERCENT REDUCTION IN ATTACK DURATION

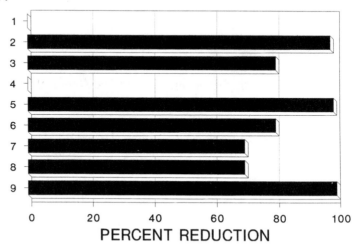

FIG. 1. Percent reduction in duration of hemiplegic attacks during treatment with flunarizine. Patients 1 and 4 did not show any change in their attacks.

complete cessation of attacks and this response has persisted for almost 2 years (Fig. 1). The family noted that the child improved in all aspects of her development during this period.

The frequency of the hemiplegic attacks however, decreased in only 3 of the 9 patients studied (Fig. 3). The average decrease was of the order of 55% in these patients. One had an increase in the number of attacks while receiving the drug.

Flunarizine seems to alter the outcome of the condition in some patients but this is difficult to document. Flunarizine is a bifluorated piperazine that selectively binds to nitrendipine calcium, alpha-adrenergic, serotonin, dopamine, and histamine sites, and inhibits intracellular calcium transfer (3,4). It has a long half-life of 19 days and a steady-state level is reached in approximately 6 weeks. The drug has also been used as a wide spectrum anticonvulsant. In several studies it has been shown to be a beneficial adjuvant with improvement in seizures 38% (5). However it has been used primarily as a prophylactic agent for the prevention of migraine and has been estimated to reduce headache frequency by 70% (6).

Casaer et al. (7) in the European cooperative study treated 12 children in an open-label and double blind flunarizine trial. All seemed to respond favorably with reduction of the hemiplegic attacks but there were relapses. The authors stressed that this

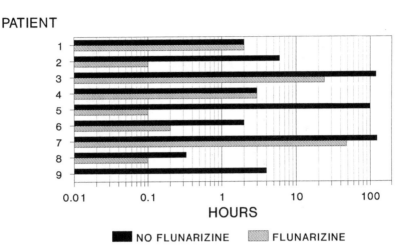

FIG. 2. Logarithmic plot of the duration of hemiplegic attacks (in hours) for each patient, comparing duration with and without flunarizine treatment. For most patients there was a decrease in duration when they were treated with flunarizine. Patient 9 had no further attacks after treatment with flunarizine was started.

was the first medication that showed some beneficial response. Our experience with this agent was similar. Only one patient had complete control of the hemiplegic attacks and subsequently also demonstrated improvement in developmental milestones. Most had an impressive reduction in the duration of the hemiplegic attacks but the frequency decreased only in a minority. There were no obvious side effects, in particular no abnormal weight gain or new abnormal movements. Patient 3 discontinued flunarizine because the attacks became more severe though the intervals between them were more prolonged.

In conclusion flunarizine has been shown to be beneficial in this disease. In one patient the hemiplegic attacks ceased completely. The plasma concentrations are known to vary considerably. Patients often take concomitant anticonvulsants that can enhance the hepatic metabolism of flunarizine and result in inadequate plasma levels. Measurement of flunarizine plasma levels might be helpful in optimizing treatment (8). Putative sites of action of this compound are not only smooth muscle vasculature but also neuronal calcium channels. It is known to have an affinity for several central nervous system binding sites. The exact site of action in patients with alternating hemiplegia however remains unknown.

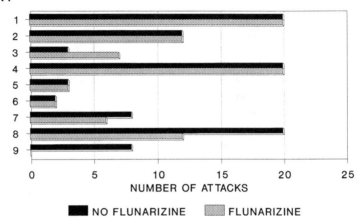

FIG. 3. Histogram showing the number of attacks per month prior to and during flunarizine treatment. Most patients did not show a decrease in frequency when treated with flunarizine.

REFERENCES

1. Casaer P, Azou M. Flunarizine in alternating hemiplegia in childhood. *Lancet* 1984;2:579.
2. Andermann F, Silver K, St. Hilaire MH. Paroxysmal alternating hemiplegia of childhood: Treatment with flunarizine and other agents. *Neurology* 1986;36:327(abst).
3. Snyder S, Reynolds I. Calcium Antagonist Drugs. *N Engl J Med* 1985;313:995–1002.
4. Levsen J, Gommeren W. In vitro receptor binding profile of drugs used in migraine. In: Amerg WK, Van Neuten JD, Wanguier A, eds. *The pharmacological basis of migraine therapy*. London: Pitman; 1984:256–266.
5. Binnie CD, de Beukelaar F, Meijer J, et al. Open dose-ranging trial of flunarizine as add-on therapy in epilepsy. *Epilepsia* 1985;26:424–428.
6. Martinez Lage JM, Olesen J, Sjaastad O. Flunarizine in the treatment of migraine: State of the art. *Cephalalgia* 1988;8(Suppl 8):1–40.
7. Casaer P. Flunarizine in alternating hemiplegia in childhood. An international study in 12 children. *Neuropediatrics* 1987;18:191–195.
8. Kapetanovic IM, Torchin CD, Kupferberg HJ, et al. Pharmacokinetic profile of flunarizine after single and multiple dosing in epileptic patients receiving comedication. *Epilepsia* 1988;29:770–774.

Alternating Hemiplegia of Childhood, edited by
Frederick Andermann, Jean Aicardi, and Federico Vigevano,
Raven Press, Ltd., New York © 1995.

25

Treatment of Alternating Hemiplegia of Childhood in Japan

Observations Based on Experience with 23 Patients

Norio Sakuragawa

Department of Inherited Metabolic Diseases, National Institute of Neuroscience, National Center for Neurology and Psychiatry, 4-1-1, Ogawahigashi-cho, Kodaira, Tokyo 187, Japan.

In 1984, Casaer and Azou (1) described dramatic improvement in a patient with alternating hemiplegia of childhood (AHC) after flunarizine treatment. Since then, flunarizine has been used in Japan. According to a large Japanese cooperative study of 23 cases of AHC (2), flunarizine was effective in decreasing the frequency and severity of attacks in three-fourths of the patients. Another Ca antagonist, nicardipine hydrochloride, was reported to be effective in one patient in reducing the frequency of hemiplegic attacks. Anticonvulsants such as phenobarbital, diphenylhydantoin, valproic acid, carbamazepine, and acetazolamide were ineffective. However, intravenous diazepam was effective in treating an acute episode of hemiplegia, which disappeared on awakening from the sleep induced by the diazepam injection. Clonazepam and diazepam given orally showed some benefit in reducing the severity and frequency of hemiplegic attacks in 5 patients out of the 23 Japanese children. Extended follow-up will be necessary to confirm any alteration of the long-term clinical course of the disease. Several other drugs have been used, but had no beneficial effect: cinepazine maleate, propranolol hydrochloride, papaverine hydrochloride, pentoxifylline, clonidine hydrochloride, fluribiprofen, L-dopa, aspirin, ubera, and ATP.

Interestingly, sleep terminates the hemiplegic episodes. Chloral hydrate suppositories seem to abolish the acute hemiplegia by having the child fall asleep (3). Trichlorethyl phosphate monosodium given rectally led to sleep and cessation of hemiplegia in one Japanese patient (2).

REFERENCES

1. Casaer P, Azou M. Flunarizine in alternating hemiplegia in childhood *Lancet* 1984;II:579.
2. Sakuragawa N. Alternating hemiplegia in childhood: 23 cases in Japan. *Brain Dev* 1992;14:283–288.
3. Siemes H, Casaer P. Alternierende Hemiplegie des Kindesalters. Klinischer Bericht und SPECT-Studie. *Monatsschr Kinderheilkd* 1988;136:467–470.

Alternating Hemiplegia of Childhood, edited by
Frederick Andermann, Jean Aicardi, and Federico Vigevano,
Raven Press, Ltd., New York © 1995.

26

Treatment of Alternating Hemiplegia of Childhood: The Effect of Haloperidol

John Wilson

*Department of Neurology, Great Ormond Street Hospital for Children, Great Ormond
Street, London WC1N 3JH, England.*

At the time that Casaer and colleagues published their letter to the *Lancet* describing a dramatically favorable response to flunarizine (1), Salmon and I were preparing a case report describing the serendipitous observation by Salmon which I confirmed in another patient, that haloperidol was also dramatically beneficial in the symptomatic treatment of alternating hemiplegia. Attacks ceased for an extended period (2).

Unlike flunarizine, haloperidol has not been submitted to a double blind controlled trial, but as in the case of flunarizine later experience has shown that it is not a panacea, although some patients seem to be consistently benefitted, with attack frequency reduced by 50% or more. Using a starting dose of 0.5 mg twice daily in the very young, the amount can be increased gradually as necessary and as tolerated to 4 mg daily in two divided doses, administering orphenadrine concurrently if there are dyskinetic side-effects.

Because of the precipitating effect of excitement I have given some patients propranolol but without any convincing benefit. Anticonvulsants are indicated only when there is clear evidence of a concurrent epileptic disorder.

Although it could be argued that the early favorable observations with both flunarizine and haloperidol were placebo effects, I find this difficult to accept because I have not seen similar responses to other drugs such as antiepileptic drugs and propranolol. It may be of significance that flunarizine and haloperidol are similar structurally and their beneficial effects, albeit transient, may have therapeutic and biochemical significance as the nature of this fascinating disorder is better understood.

REFERENCES

1. Casaer P, Azou M. Flunarizine in alternating hemiplegia in childhood. *Lancet* 1984;2:579
2. Salmon MA, Wilson J. Drugs for alternating hemiplegia. *Lancet* 1984;2:980.

Alternating Hemiplegia of Childhood, edited by
Frederick Andermann, Jean Aicardi, and Federico Vigevano,
Raven Press, Ltd., New York © 1995.

27

Rectal Chloral Hydrate for Treatment of Alternating Hemiplegia of Childhood

Hartmut Siemes

Department of Pediatrics, Rittberg-Krankenhaus, D-12205, Berlin, Germany.

Despite the favorable influence of flunarizine on frequency, duration, and severity of hemiplegic episodes (2,4,5) most children suffer from ongoing attacks. It would be very helpful to have a drug by which the parents could block an attack immediately at occurrence so that the patient can go on with his usual activities. Rectal chloral hydrate seems to be such a promising drug.

Rectal chloral hydrate is usually employed as a sedative and as an anticonvulsant in children. In therapeutic doses it has little effect on respiration and blood pressure. It is very rapidly reduced to trichlorethanol (half-life of a few minutes), a central-depressant metabolite (plasma half-life from 4 to 12 hours), conjugated with glucuronic acid, and finally excreted in the urine. Undesirable CNS effects are malaise and ataxia; however, the hangover is less common than with barbiturates and benzodiazepines (3).

In a first trial 1 to 2 tubes of rectal chloral hydrate (one tube containing 600 mg dissolved in sesame-oil) were used in an infant for induction of sleep, since interruption of hemiplegias by sleep is a characteristic clinical feature of the disease. Usually the patient fell asleep for hours, with no hemiplegia after waking. As the child grew older, rectal chloral hydrate led to disappearance of the hemiplegias without causing sleep (6). No side-effects were noted, if only one half to one tube was used; two tubes caused sedation and ataxia.

Meanwhile two further children with alternating hemiplegia have also been treated with rectal chloral hydrate. All three children met the diagnostic criteria as outlined by Aicardi (1). They all received the drug at least 100 times. It was found effective in all children. However, it only stopped the hemiplegia, if it was applied shortly (within a few minutes) after the onset of an attack. In one of the three patients the influence of chloral hydrate on the appearance of attacks of hemiplegia had been well documented by the mother. With a total of 76 applications over a 9-month period the ratio of effective to ineffective interventions was 2.5:1. If only one half to one tube was used there were no side-effects; the children could go on with their usual activities. In case of a complete failure of one rectal dose the administration of another dose was ineffective. However, if there was an initial effect and the hemiplegia recurred after some time the repeated application of chloral hydrate remained effective. When a bilateral attack started this drug generally caused a change to unilateral manifestations. This could be observed even if the attack had persisted for some time. The company which sells chloral hydrate in tubes had used sesame oil as a solvent for some time. Since the manufacturing firm had problems with the stability of their product they first switched over to peanut oil and finally to medium-chain tryglicerides. All parents made the observation that rectal chloral hydrate in sesame oil was most effective. In the child in whom the effect of rectal chloral hydrate was best documented, the success ratio of effective to ineffective applications using sesame oil was 4:1 compared to peanut oil with 1:1. During the last 6 months we have been using another solvent (600 mg chloral hydrate added to 2,400 mg distilled water containing 15% ethanol) with even more success, since this preparation acts much more rapidly and more reliably.

An important factor influencing the effectiveness of rectal chloral hydrate are the accompanying circumstances. It is much easier to block an attack if the child is calm and in relaxed surroundings than in a loud and turbulent situation. In that case the child should be brought into a quiet room or into a quiet corner of a room where the rectal chloral hydrate is administered.

Rectal chloral hydrate has been used for several years in these children who are now between 4 and 6 years of age. Short-term side-effects can be avoided using a low dose (½ to 1 tube seems to be appropriate for this age group). However, we do not know anything about possible long-term positive or negative effects of this drug.

REFERENCES

1. Aicardi J. Alternating hemiplegia of childhood. *Int Pediatr* 1987;2:115–119.
2. Casaer P, Azou M. Flunarizine in alternating hemiplegia in childhood. *Lancet* 1984;2:579.
3. Chloral hydrate. In: Goodman S, Rall TW, Murad F, eds. *Goodman and Gilman's, The pharmacological basis of therapeutics*, Seventh ed. New York: MacMillan; 1985:360–362.
4. Curatolo P, Cusmai R. Drugs for alternating hemiplegia. *Lancet* 1984;2:980.
5. Casaer P. Flunarizine in alternating hemiplegia in childhood. An international study in 12 children. *Neuropediatrics* 1987;18:191–195.
6. Siemes H. Rectal chloral hydrate for alternating hemiplegia of childhood. *Dev Med Child Neurol* 1990;32:927–931.

Conclusions

Alternating Hemiplegia of Childhood, edited by
Frederick Andermann, Jean Aicardi, and Federico Vigevano,
Raven Press, Ltd., New York © 1995.

28

Alternating Hemiplegia of Childhood: An Overview

*Jean Aicardi, **Marie Bourgeois, †Lucia Fusco,
†Federico Vigevano, ‡Kenneth Silver, and ‡Frederick Andermann

*Institute of Child Health, University of London, Mecklenburgh Square,
London WC1N 2AP, England; **Hôpital des Enfants Malades, 149 rue de Sèvre,
75743, Paris Cedex 15, France; †Section of Neurophysiology,
"Bambino Gesù" Children's Hospital, Piazza S. Onofrio, 4 00165 Rome, Italy; and
‡Departments of Neurology, Neurosurgery, and Pediatrics, McGill University,
Montreal Neurological Hospital and Institute, 3801 University Street,
Montreal, Quebec H3A 2B4, Canada. Montreal Children's Hospital, 2300 Tupper Street,
Montreal, Quebec, H3H IP3, Canada.*

The saga of alternating hemiplegia of childhood (AHC) began 23 years ago with the initial description by Simon Verret and John Steele of eight children with a remarkable clinical picture of episodes of weakness of one side of the body associated with other symptoms. With the benefit of hindsight, it now seems that several of these children had "classical" hemiplegic migraine but three of them had the distinctive features of AHC as we understand it today.

In the 20 odd years that have elapsed since, the delineation of the condition has been refined and it has become clear that AHC is a disease in its own right and that a number of variants and related disorders exist.

Several investigators have confirmed the observations of Verret and Steele and added to their description a series of bizarre paroxysmal manifestations, that include nystagmus and other oculomotor abnormalities, tonic or dystonic attacks, and respiratory and autonomic changes. The secondary emergence of developmental retardation and of nonparoxysmal neurological symptoms in affected children, especially ataxia and choreoathetotic movements, has been recognized as a constant feature. It has thus become clear that nonparoxysmal features and a cohort of unusual clinical symptoms associated with the hemiplegic attacks are more characteristic of AHC than the hemiplegias themselves and separate the condition from hemiplegic migraine though a possible relationship between the two conditions remains a possibility.

AHC, as defined today, comprises a core of stereotyped features so striking that its recognition is obvious when the condition is known. The first manifestations are usually tonic attacks and paroxysmal nystagmus rather than hemiplegias, and these appear early in life, sometimes even in the neonatal period. At this stage, the occurrence of brief tonic paroxysms, usually involving one side of the body, almost inevitably suggests a seizure disorder, the more so as the dystonic episodes are often associated with a vibratory tremor of the extended limbs and followed by hemiparesis, often first regarded as Todd's paralysis. Abnormal eye movements are quite suggestive of AHC, especially monocular nystagmus. Recent work has shown that, at least in some cases, nystagmus is part of a complex oculomotor disturbance, closely resembling internuclear ophthalmoplegia or the "one-and-a-half syndrome" (lateral gaze palsy to one side with contralateral palsy of adduction as a result of a lesion involving the pontine paramedian reticular formation and the longitudinal fasciculus on the same side), which points to brainstem involvement at the level of the pons. However, other ocular disturbances (e.g., vertical nystagmus or large amplitude movements of the globe in multiple directions) may also be found.

The hemiplegic episodes, even though they are not usually the first symptom, appear before 18 months, and almost always during the first year of life. The hemiplegic attacks have unusual characteristics: they may occur suddenly, often precipitated by affective stimuli, and be preceded by screaming and fussiness; they vary in intensity from one moment to the next; they are usually not associated with pyramidal tract signs but are characterized by changes in muscle tone. Bilateral episodes of weakness and tonic modifications are a most remarkable and typical feature of AHC. Few, if any, conditions lead to such attacks alternating with hemiplegic episodes. Bilateral attacks can be the sole manifestation of a paroxysmal episode or they may occur at the time when a hemiplegic attack switches to the opposite side. These paroxysms can be very frightening, since they are often accompanied by respiratory distress and other autonomic disturbances.

Another characteristic feature of AHC is the disappearance of all abnormalities when the child falls asleep. This symptom is of such diagnostic importance that specific enquiry about the effect of sleep is essential. In prolonged episodes, there is often recurrence of the paralysis on awakening but there is first a 10 to 20 minute period of freedom from paralysis. Many parents take advantage of this gap in order to feed the children. Such a history is often volunteered by the parents and is highly suggestive of the diagnosis. The importance of sleep in leading to the disappearance of paroxysmal motor phenomena suggests that mechanisms underlying the sleep-waking cycle are in some way involved, not only in causing the paroxysms to cease but also in causing them to appear. Sleep has an analogous role in other disorders. In some migraine syndromes attacks cease during sleep; in some dystonias, particularly in Segawa's syndrome, and in certain forms of juvenile Parkinson's disease sleep leads to striking changes in the symptoms such as for instance a reduction in rigidity.

In alternating hemiplegia, it is not clear whether the hemiplegic attack itself triggers sleep. Neither is it clear whether these patients have a normal sleep/waking cycle. Often at the onset of a hemiplegic attack phenomena resembling the onset of sleep occur: yawning, diffuse loss of tone, and a tendency to lean for support or dropping of the head. Even the hemiplegic paroxysmal phenomena themselves could be interpreted as a sleep-like state: the prodromal symptoms such as yawning, followed by hypotonia, and eventually loss of tone accompanied on the electroencephalogram by low-amplitude theta discharges are features typical of REM sleep.

The attacks of alternating hemiplegia also resemble cataplectic attacks, in which a complete loss of muscular tone coexists with a normal state of consciousness. However, patients with alternating hemiplegia show a normal pattern of sleep onset in contrast to the abnormal patterns found in patients with narcolepsy or cataplexy.

The paralytic episodes recur at variable intervals and have a variable duration. They may recur for many years even though they often tend to become less complex or more purely hemiplegic. After variable periods, it becomes evident that the children do not progress normally and most are left with increasingly obvious and severe mental retardation. They also become ataxic, and choreoathetosis of variable severity further compounds the overall disability. AHC is therefore a severe and often malignant disease which is not usually compatible with an independent life and may, in some cases, lead to death from pulmonary complications.

The disorder may appear in a normal infant although the young age at onset makes it difficult to be categoric about this. Probably, more often, it supervenes in an infant who has initially slow development. Hypotonia before the onset of paroxysms has been repeatedly reported.

A major, unanswered question is whether the disease is progressive or whether the disability merely becomes more evident with increasing age. Our current impression is that there may be early deterioration during the first two years of the course, followed by a period of relative stability. However, progressive deterioration is not easily excluded and a possible role of the acute episodes in leading to a decline in brain function must be considered. This applies particularly to bilateral episodes that are not infrequently followed by a marked regression of previously acquired skills. Although affected infants seem to recover from such attacks, no detailed study of cognitive and performance levels before and after acute episodes is available. Thus the significance of the acute paroxysms and their role in leading to delayed development remains to be established. This issue is of practical importance, as prevention of the acute episodes may become possible when better drugs are available.

Seizures occur in 50% of patients with AHC. Seizures hardly ever occur as presenting symptoms; neither are they particularly severe in the early years of the disease. They may occur in close relationship to a hemiplegic attack. How the two syndromes relate to one another however is far from clear. The seizures are predominantly partial, in many patients occur frequently, and they may manifest as status epilepticus late in the course of the disease. This association implies that cortical involvement may be related or secondary to a disturbance in subcortical structures that seem to be primarily involved in causing the symptoms of AHC.

AHC is such a distinctive disorder that it can be separated relatively easily from a number of other diseases that may be responsible for alternating hemiplegia. Vascular disorders such as A-V malformations and multiple emboli or thromboses rarely if ever raise a problem in differential diagnosis. A few rare cases, such as those of patients with repeated episodes of transient hemiplegia associated with Osler-

Weber-Rendu disease or with cutis marmorata congenita, may more closely resemble AHC. Pyruvate dehydrogenase deficiency has led to recurrent attacks of alternating hemiplegia in at least one patient. Metabolic diseases (e.g., Leigh's disease) can feature hemiplegia but neither in vascular nor in metabolic conditions has the full spectrum of the bizarre paroxysmal symptoms typical of AHC been observed. Indeed, the term AHC is in some respects a misnomer since the hemiplegias are often not the most distinctive feature of the condition.

A major issue concerning the etiology of alternating hemiplegia is its relationship with migraine. The earliest descriptions and most of the ones since, led to the suspicion of vascular involvement, perhaps because of the traditional neurological experience with hemiplegia due to vascular disease but also because of the clinical symptomatology which suggested a hemispheral etiology. The hypotonia and the early dystonic attacks did not attract a great deal of attention at that time, and since most children were young, the eventual development of athetosis or dystonia was not very obvious.

The presence of a family history of migraine is ubiquitous in some series of patients and less frequent in others. It is likely that these differences are more in the eye of the beholder or the diagnostician, than in fact. There is no comparable incongruity in the description of any of the other clinical features of AHC, the response to medication, or the outcome. Thus we may conclude that these differences may relate to variability in diagnostic criteria based on cultural and other perspectives rather than on differences between the Western European, British, Japanese, or North American populations where large series of patients with alternating hemiplegia have been described.

The patients themselves are miserable and unhappy before and during the attacks and in small children this is difficult to interpret. As they get older stomach or head pain are mentioned but the children are not terribly specific. In teenagers, especially in occasional brighter ones, a history may be obtained suggestive of a migrainous march but such observations are rare (see Chapter 2; L.B.P. Stephenson, *personal communication*, 1991).

Although AHC has been frequently regarded as a form of hemiplegic migraine, there are enough differences between the two syndromes to consider them distinct conditions. Furthermore, hemiplegic migraine is usually not associated with progressive deficit. Migraine coma, or hemiplegic migraine with peduncular hallucinosis is emerging as a specific entity and the reason for the associated progressive neurological syndrome, consisting of ataxia or tremor and abnormal eye movements is not clear. Dominantly inherited hemiplegic migraine may also be associated with vascular malformations such as the Osler-Weber-Rendu syndrome and migraine is a common finding associated with familial cavernous angioma. In these conditions it may perhaps be related to abnormal vascular permeability. Hemiplegic migraine rarely has its onset before two years of age and does not feature tonic attacks, oculomotor abnormalities, or mental retardation.

Alternating hemiplegia is not the only instance where a family history of migraine is associated with a malignant neurological disorder. In our experience the patients with sporadic MELAS syndrome have all had a family background of migraine. They do not have any of the point mutations identified so far in familial cases, and the reason for the decompensation of a single member in a family with many migrainous individuals has not been explained.

The relationship to migraine is suggestive also in benign familial nocturnal alternating hemiplegia. In the family reported in this volume the family history of migraine was both clear and striking and in the siblings with this entity mentioned by Verret and Steele migraine was present in the family as well. There are unfortunately no descriptions of long-term follow-up in that sibship. The occurrence in siblings in both families is another important feature distinguishing these patients from those with the now classical sporadic variety. The onset out of sleep and the lack of deterioration seem characteristic, but longer follow-up is required.

Is AHC a single disease? The homogeneous clinical presentation strongly supports this assumption and patients reported from various parts of the world (viz., Western Europe, North America, and Japan) are remarkably similar. In the past few years, however, there have been reports of children with clinical pictures departing in one or more major points from the usual stereotyped pattern. The children with hypotonia and paroxysmal dystonic episodes precipitated by excitement, and which in one child were followed by the late appearance of hemiplegic attacks, choreoathetosis, and an excellent response to flunarizine illustrate this. Benign familial nocturnal alternating hemiplegia is so closely related to AHC that it was initially thought to be the same condition. However, the emergence of hemiplegias exclusively out of sleep, the normal cognitive development, and the familial character, represent major differences that justify setting apart these rare patients.

A familial form of AHC has also been reported by Mikati and collaborators. The clinical manifestations are quite similar to those of the usual sporadic cases and these patients fulfill the criteria for inclusion as AHC. There are, however, subtle differences: the most notable is the lesser severity of the autosomal dominant form. Some affected individuals in Mikati's family remained normal up to the age of 3 years, managed to lead relatively independent lives, and to procreate. Whether these differences are sufficient to define a special variant will have to await recognition of further affected families. If the relation to the disease of a translocation between chromosomes 3 and 9 found in four of the five subjects in Mikati's family, is confirmed, this may provide a clue to the etiology of the condition. Further karyotype studies should be considered, even in sporadic cases.

The magnetic resonance spectroscopic abnormalities in children with alternating hemiplegia suggest the presence of mitochondrial dysfunction. However, these abnormalities may fluctuate. In a child with the nocturnal familial form abnormalities were present early in life when the attacks were more frequent and more severe. The pattern returned to normal several years later when the attacks were less frequent. Clearly, studies in more patients as well as serial examinations are required to clarify this aspect.

The present therapy of AHC is far from satisfactory and the effect of treatment on long-term outcome is uncertain. Multiple trials of antiepileptic and antimigraine drugs have generally been ineffective. Some parents, however, are convinced that discontinuation of phenytoin increases the frequency and severity of attacks. Some positive results have been reported with haloperidol and chloral hydrate. Flunarizine, a calcium channel blocking agent, has been most extensively tested and clearly reduces the severity and duration of the hemiplegic episodes in many patients. It has however relatively little effect on the frequency of the episodes. Not much is known about its mechanism of action in AHC. Moreover, we do not understand why the drug is completely ineffective in some patients, why it seems to be immediately effective in the face of a very long half-life, why its efficacy is only partial, and why the effect wears off in some children. We clearly need other, better drugs but testing their efficacy will require cooperative studies since the incidence of the disease is too low for sufficient patients to be collected and treated in any one center. Long-term results of any new therapy will, in all likelihood be difficult to evaluate just as was the case with flunarizine.

From the review of the classical syndrome as defined by Aicardi and of its variants and other syndromes reported here it becomes clear that alternation of hemiplegia and the tendency to the development of bilateral attacks is shared by this whole group of disorders. The assessment of the effect of sleep on other paroxysmal movement disorders, particularly dystonia, is likely to provide further information. The absence of pyramidal lesions and pyramidal deficits in AHC even after a great number of episodes is striking. The negative motor phenomena suggest primarily subcortical involvement. The basic mechanisms of alternating hemiplegia remain open to interpretation, though the clinical features clearly pointed to a multisystem disorder, involving the motor system (hypotonia, hemiplegia, and dystonia), the oculomotor system (interictal nystagmus, ictal gaze paralysis), and the associative areas (the majority of the patients have cognitive deficits).

When AHC is suspected, it is essential to try to reach a specific diagnosis and to distinguish between the different entities we have illustrated in this volume since they may have different etiologies and prognosis despite some clinical resemblance.

The suggestion of an abnormality of energy metabolism and of mitochondrial dysfunction in patients with AHC in the absence of demonstrable structural abnormalities encourages us to continue investigations in that area.

Subject Index